EAR CANDLING AND OTHER TREATMENTS

FOR EAR, NOSE AND THROAT PROBLEMS

This book is dedicated to my mother, Anne, without whose
help and support this book would not have been possible.

CONTENTS

Chapter 10: Continued

Diagrams

Colour Plates (between pages 89-90)

Author carrying out an ear candling treatment
Equipment needed for an ear candling treatment
Different types of residue found in used ear candles
Examples of different types of ear candles
Labelled parts of the auricle
Labelled parts of the ear
Examples of hearing tests using a tuning fork
The Aurex 3 plus tinnitus therapy device
A cochlear implant in place
A Hearing Dog for the Deaf in action
Example of the use of ear protection

ACKNOWLEDGEMENTS

In life, we all need others to either learn from or to help us progress as citizens of the world so that we can leave it a better place by our endeavours.

The first person I must thank is my mother Anne who has given me much love and care through my life. Without my mother's help and encouragement this book would not have been brought into existence - a true 'Angel' in more than one sense. My late father Jack, who loved the Candles treatment, is probably looking down on me from above taking his snuff and smiling as usual. My partner Karen and her father Norman have put up with me now for over ten years and have made me smile at the strangest things. Norman was able to help with some photographs and Karen, who is a prize winning artist, is my wizard with the book illustrations and also the work with my PC. Karen's twin brother Ian also took some photographs and brought the production and design of the book up to speed and made it ready for Paul Jones, Gary Williams and the excellent organisation at Welshpool Printing Group. Praise should also be directed to Lucy who was my enthusiastic model for the ear candling photograph on the book cover, a real pleasure to work with. Peter Love and Gary Bailey at Peter Love PR and Advertising helped greatly with the minutae of the pre and launch marketing of the book.

I was pleased to call on the services of a number of people who were able to furnish me with information about their therapies or remedial equipment which can be used. Robin Butterfield, DO, ND, Doctor of Osteopathy and Remedial Masseur who is greatly experienced and who practices in Ludlow supplied me with background information about osteopathy and made useful comments on this part of the book. John and Sonya Downes provided me with information about hearing enhancement devices and equipment for the Deaf and hard of hearing based mainly on their experience as volunteers in the Audiology Hearing Advisory Unit at Ashford Hospital, Middlesex.

Tina Griffith, Gill Berry and Paul Siroky of the Visual Interpreting and Communication Service in Shropshire (VISS) who are based in Shrewsbury very kindly gave up some of their time to talk about their work with the disabled community and then commented on the sections of the book dealing with hearing enhancement and communication services which are available. Tina Pascal from Midsomer Norton kindly enlightened me about Health Kinesiology and helped me with this section in the book.

David Thomas and Eric Churchyard of Shrewsbury Medical Limited provided the background to the new 'Aurex 3 plus Tinnitus Therapy Device' which is designed to ameliorate the suffering of people unfortunate to have the condition. I am pleased to support this company which manufactures, services and supplies general medical equipment. Louise Betz supplied a lot of information about cochlear implants which her company, Advanced Bionics UK Ltd, supplies. The video this company supplied to me 'Cecilia's Story' which tells the story of how a brave little girl had an implant fitted and the improvements it made to her life is truly inspiring.

As a dog owner myself I had a wonderful treat when I visited the headquarters of the charity Hearing Dogs for Deaf People. My visit was organised by Nikki Wright their Press and PR Officer and as well as having a tour of the facilities I saw Ben Sargeant a trainer working with Samba a most intelligent spaniel recruit of theirs. Nikki also kindly suggested improvements to the section in the book about the work of the charity.

Grant Robson and Emily Richardson of the Deafness Research UK (formerly the Defeating Deafness (The Hearing Research Trust)) charity helped me with enquiries about research being carried out in the UK about glue ear and tinnitus and also sent me publicity information which could be used in my video and I was pleased to have recently donated a speaking fee to their charity. Nicola Woodgate very kindly sent me some information about Goldenhar Syndrome and her charity provides valuable support for sufferers of this rare condition and their families.

Whenever I visited the RNID Library which is situated within the Royal National Throat, Nose and Ear Hospital, Gray's Inn Road, London I was fortunate to be helped by Mary Plackett the then Librarian. She worked very efficiently but more importantly she made me, and all the other visitors, very welcome to her treasure trove of relevant medical information. For anyone interested in learning about ENT matters this library is a 'must' to visit.

To all those organisers who have been brave enough to invite and reinvite me back to teach my accredited courses for them I would particularly thank Cathy Hamouy of Complementary-Therapies School Gerrards Cross; Susan Prentice, Margaret Atkins and their colleagues at the Essex group of the Association of Reflexology; Susie and Howard Bradley at the Abbey School of Therapeutic Massage, Bexleyheath; Tina Pascal, Phil and her colleagues at the Positive Living Centre Midsomer Norton; Sue and Rick Ager at the Ager School of Aromatherapy Colchester; Louise Searles at the Phoenix School Chelmsford; Jenin Burton and Jennifer Clarke at Bromley College; Barbara Jackson who was at Bedminster College Bristol and all her colleagues; Fran Keen and all the therapists doing wonderful work at the Broadway Lodge Weston-super-Mare; Pauline-Morgan Jones in Whitchurch Bristol; Trish Lewis in Yate; Myrtle Turner, Nina Foot, Jean Jones, Winnie Vettraino and all the other members of the Scottish Institute of Reflexology who made me so welcome one special teaching weekend in Edinburgh and Elizabeth and Bob Armstrong and Renni at the Angel Centre, Gateshead.

I have learnt much from all my amazing students whom I think of as my extended 'family' - teaching must be a two way process and I have learnt a great deal from them. They have come from all fields of therapy interest but a special group who expanded my knowledge was the nursing tutors and back up staff at the Primary Ear Care Centre, Kiveton Park, Sheffield led by Linda Mills. It was through her kind offices that I was invited to be part of a study day where I successfully demonstrated the Ear Candles treatment to 150 NHS nursing staff. I learnt about the Primary Ear Care Centre and its excellent nurse training from Hilary Harkin who as well as being one of my students has written the 'Guidance on Ear Care', for the Action on ENT Steering Board, which has been endorsed by the Royal Colleges of General Practitioners and Nurses, the Primary Ear Care Centre and the Medical Devices Agency.

Hilary is an excellent example of a nurse dedicated to her profession. Some of my other students merit special mention and these include Sharon McDade who has helped me run courses in Devon; Barbara Perry who assisted me in Hampshire; Kareth Paterson who is now teaching a family and friends Candling course in Hillingdon and whom I first met at the Iver Nature Study Centre which is well worth a visit; Jacqui Hingerton who is wonderful well grounded lady who together with Alaine and Carolyn Biggs and Shilpa Patel formed a close knit group that I took from Usui Reiki 1 to Reiki Master level in three magical weekends at Carolyn's House.

I have been lucky enough to encounter some generous genuine people in my travels and of these perhaps my good friend Dr Neville Sutton is paramount. I have known Neville, who is now retired, for over twenty years since I ran a rehabilitation gym at his GP practice in Harlington. He embodies all that is best in a GP - caring and very sympathetic with time for everyone. I value very highly our friendship and the advice which he gives me.

Another remarkable person is Sheila Bennett with whom I forged a great friendship in London and who as well as being an expert in her therapy field has a wonderful garden at her home in London. When I studied reflexology with Sandra Watson in Maidenhead I was not to know then that we would develop our relationship to such an extent that I would become a Reiki Master under her tutelage, discover that my angel is called Seth and that my first Ear Candle teaching would be done in her front room. She is a great deal of fun and has a charming family; I have much to thank her for. Another person who has shaped my thinking is Jack Weller, a wonderful hypnotherapist based in Buckinghamshire under whom I studied. Jack is excellent at his job, incredibly perceptive and is a true man of peace and love.

Teaching my courses was encouraged by Patricia Collis and Lesley Alexander at the Evreham Education Centre, Iver, Buckinghamshire and their support was backed up by the Buckinghamshire Educational authority which financially supported me on my City and Guilds teaching course. I will always remember Harvey at Evreham who was always helping me when the photocopier became jammed. In the time that I have been teaching the ear candles therapy I have had a great deal of help from Raj Vora and his team at Revital in Ruislip who import and distribute the candles which I use. I always enjoy visiting his shop and nosing among all the products, books and gadgets that are on offer.

I will mention Tony Allwood in the foreword but I would like to thank all the members of the BNI chapter in Shrewsbury, where I am a member, for their friendship and help. I would recommend anyone starting up in business or moving to a new area to work to consider joining a local networking group such as BNI. Two other people to be singled out are Allison Timmins who is a caring lady with a love of animals and Keith Higgins who has helped my business thinking and philosophy.

Hopefully, with my varied therapy work and this book I will live up to the BNI motto 'Givers Gain'; a philosophy I would recommend to therapists and all others.

FOREWORD

When I first thought about writing this book about three years ago it was simply going to cover and accompany the Ear Candling therapy which I have taught on my accredited courses to over 1,600 students to date (November 2005) all over the United Kingdom. The scope of the book grew like Topsy and everytime I thought that I had finished it another nugget of information about the ear, nose and throat and their problems and treatment came my way and cried out to be included in the pages that you are about to read.

Although there are general books available on individual ear, nose or throat conditions I thought that it would be useful to bring many of the main conditions with some of the rarer ones together. As this book is aimed at diverse groups including therapists and the general public I thought that instead of cluttering up the pages with detailed references I would usually include this information in the body of the text. If any reader would like to receive further information this can be sourced through my email address pressuredown@tesco.net or on the courses I teach. Any repitition of information is meant to be a reinforcement of learning for the reader.

I hope that the reader will find the chapter on ear candling of interest. I hope that I have explained this therapy quite clearly and hopefully it will answer many questions about this controversial treatment which are often asked by my students and elsewhere. I should say that my views have changed over the years especially since I now have the ability to check the ear canal and my commissioned research which has analysed the contents of candle filters after they have been used. It should be added that views about this therapy are mixed and several organisations including the British Tinnitus Association are not supportive of it at all and have distanced themselves from it. The biggest change in this edition of the book is the alteration in suggested intervals between ear candling treatments which are now shorter than those recommended in the previous edition. This has come about after discussing treatment results with many other therapists.

As well as the ear candling therapy I have given a background to over twenty other complementary therapies and similar treatments which are available to the public together with suggestions about what to look for when choosing the right therapist and therapy for you. To all those therapists who are doing great healing works whose treatments have not been included I owe an apology; this has not meant to be a slight on your skills and expertise but simply the fact that I could not include every treatment as this would be a basis for a separate book even longer than this one.

As a complementary therapist I thought that something which would try to bridge the divide which has grown up and hopefully is now being broken down between conventional medicine and complementary therapy is a good thing. Each field has something to offer and it is important for the patient or client to be offered treatment options as long as those being offered are safe and potentially helpful.

My interest in therapies to help ear, nose and throat conditions was stimulated by the fact that I have learnt at first hand about the problems caused by different degrees of hearing impairment, tinnitus and Ménière's Disease from those around me. If anything can be done to help them and the many millions who suffer like them this must be a worthwhile thing. I guess that my interest in massage, which was the first complementary therapy in which I qualified, was first seen at the tender age of eight when I was paid six old pennies to massage an aunt's feet. She kept coming back for more so I think that I was doing something right!

I have always liked training and competing in different sports and as well as finishing the London Marathon three times in the early days of its life I was a reasonably good hockey player and it was in this sport that I became a qualified coach. I then supervised different types of gymnasiums including one at the old Royal Masonic Hospital, London, at a GP practice in Harlington, Middlesex where in its beginnings ice had to be chipped away from machinery in the winter and in the summer the users looked like extras from the French Foreign Legion and one in my living room. The gym users, who ranged from an Olympic gold medallist and other elite performers through to little old ladies and gentlemen and from rehab patients to fit 'Joe/ Joanna publics' often became longstanding great friends.

Having gained the ITEC qualifications in anatomy, physiology and massage and sports massage in 1987 I had to wait until 1997 to further my range of complementary therapy qualifications although in the intervening period I had attended courses as diverse as treating cancer patients with massage and using a mini- trampoline therapeutically. I am now a practitioner in Reflexology, Indian Head Massage and On-site Massage as well as being a Reiki Master. One day when visiting a health show in London I was fascinated by the sight of a lady lying on a couch with a Hopi ear candle burning in her ear. My enthusiasm was such that I was soon qualified in this therapy.

The next stage of my career development was to qualify as a teacher and this I did with the encouragement of the staff development team at the South Buckinghamshire College at Evreham, Iver. I then got my syllabus approved for both my Hopi Ear Candles and Holistic Seated Upper Body Massage courses by the Guild of Complementary Practitioners which merged with the ITEC Professionals group to become the IGPP, now Embody. My two accredited courses which I am available to teach throughout the country are now acceptable for insurance purposes by many therapy organisations. As part of my courses I offer my students an after care advice service which many of them have used.

In 2002 I moved with my family and two dogs from London to Shrewsbury, Shropshire and fell in love with my new surroundings even though I often travel hundreds of miles to teach my courses. I have received encouragement from many people including the members of the BNI networking group which meets at the ungodly hour of 6.45am once every week. Tony Allwood another BNI member and a great motorbike fan and I formed Friday Afternoon Productions and we made available a DVD 'A Guide to Ear Candling'. This was the first in a series of therapy DVDs by the author.

INTRODUCTION

The inner ear and the surrounding structures such as the nose and sinuses are extremely delicate and they usually work together in a delicate system both in isolation and in accord with each other. When one part of the whole is adversely affected by excessive noise, allergens, trauma or other causes this can have an effect on other parts of the system.

As well as there being the physical effects of imbalances which affect the individual and his/ her family, friends and colleagues there are also the social and emotional effects which can be brought about. People who suffer for instance with severe hearing impairment, Ménière's Disease, tinnitus or migraines do not usually show any external signs that mark them out as having these debilitating conditions. Many people who are deaf can find themselves locked away in their own internal environment and deafness can impinge on communication in many ways.

Helen Keller, probably the most famous deaf blind woman ever wrote movingly; 'I am just as deaf as I am blind. The problems of deafness are deeper and more complex, if not more important, than those of blindness. Deafness is a much worse misfortune. For it means the loss of the most vital stimulus - the sound of the voice that brings language, sets thoughts astir and keeps us in the intellectual company of man'.

Visually, the final scene of the 1997 film 'Cop Land' starring Sylvester Stallone as a partially deaf sheriff brought home to me the terror of suddenly becoming deaf. Stallone becomes disorientated when a pistol is fired right next to his better ear and to a hearing person such as myself the sight of dogs barking unheard or people mouthing shouting brought home what it must be like to enter the world of the Deaf.

Many famous people have suffered from conditions described in this book including Hildegard von Bingen (1098-1179) who suffered from migraine; Lewis Carroll whose slowly disappearing Cheshire Cat was probably based on disturbances associated with his classical migraine attacks; Beethoven who became deaf and Tony Benn and the Rt. Hon. Lord Ashley of Stoke who have both overcome hearing difficulties and have made great contributions to public political life in the UK and who have championed the cause of the deaf. Another famous personality associated with ENT problems was Sigmund Freud the Viennese psychoanalyst, but in his case he originally started his training as an ENT practitioner.

As we shall see later in the book problems with the ears, nose and throat have been recognised for thousands of years. Remedies going back to the ancient Assyrians are listed in the chapter on ear wax and Greek notables such as Hippocrates and Aristotle used honey as a medicinal remedy. Allergies were documented by Galen as early as the 2nd century BC.

Today there is a wide range of treatments available including advanced surgery, drugs, natural and complementary therapies and sometimes even non- intervention. Many inventions such as cochlear implants are little short of being miraculous.

Research is being conducted into a wide range of conditions such as genetic causes of deafness at birth, tinnitus and Ménière's Disease by dedicated researchers in the UK and all over the world.

Legislation to protect workers' hearing has been strengthened and hopefully this will be helped by common sense of those exposed to high noise levels at work and play. Litigation has also been influential in changing medical practice and improving worker protection. In January 2003 for example a UK civil servant was awarded substantial damages after his long term exposure to photocopier noise.

Statistics such as 1.3 million people being exposed to potentially damaging noise levels in the workplace (source:Defeating Deafness charity), 4 million people in the UK suffering from tinnitus (Defeating Deafness) and 20% of people aged 18-25 being exposed to damaging sound levels (Medical Research Council's Institute of Hearing Research, Nottingham) are extremely worrying and indicate the scale of the problem in the UK.

Equally, it is interesting that a Deaf or hard of hearing person is 2.5 times more likely to be unemployed than a hearing person (Royal National Institute for the Deaf and Hard of Hearing brief on Deafness, employment and discrimination) or that employers are 8 times more likely to employ a person with a criminal record than employ a Deaf person (RNID). Hopefully the social and economic consequences of deafness can be addressed as well as researching the causes of problems.

Hopefully, this book will help the reader to better understand the ear, nose and throat; their problems and causes and how they can be prevented and treated with the many options that are available today.

CHAPTER 1: THE EAR CANDLING THERAPY

Introduction

The Ear Candling complementary therapy has become increasingly popular in the last twenty years although it is rooted in antiquity, having been practised for hundreds if not thousands of years. The use of heat or cold in one way or another has been a natural remedy for the treatment of all manner of bodily conditions including aching muscles, carbuncles, painful teeth and gums and the common cold.

The History of Ear Candling

The ear candling therapy has many alternative titles including; 'ear coning', 'thermotherapy', 'thermal auricular therapy' and 'thermo auricular therapy'. It is possibly best known however as Hopi Ear Candling as it seems that the oldest recorded use of the Ear Candles is by the Hopi Pueblo tribe who live in the South Western part of the United States of America. Paintings of Ear Candles are in existence dating far back into history. The reasons for their use and the stories behind their use which was for both spiritual and physical purposes were not written down but painted and verbally handed down by the Shaman "holy people" of the tribe. It is probable that they were used in initiation rituals and healing ceremonies.

Some people believe that healing candles originated in the mythical ancient civilisations of Lemuria and Atlantis and that knowledge of them spread worldwide before these civilisations were engulfed in some cataclysmic disaster.

It is interesting that different ancient cultures which have survived to the modern day have used heat for healing purposes as well as providing warmth for comfort and cooking. In Mexico there are stories of cones of paper being lighted and whilst smouldering placed against the ear so that the smoke can enter the outer ear canal so causing a healing process. In the Indian sub-continent not only is there a tradition of ear cleansing from an early age with oils and wax-removing sticks but smoke is blown into the ear canal to facilitate healing. In both the sub-continent and Japan there are stories of ear cleaning booths at the roadside, although in this case implements rather than heat is used. One of my clients recounted that thirty years ago when her ear was affected by wind blowing through an open car window in Ethiopia she was later made better by the introduction of smoke into her ear by a native tribal medicine man.

In ancient Greece the ceremony of lighting the Olympic flame took on a spiritual as well as a worldly significance, this ceremony on Mount Olympus is carried on to the present day every four years.

Native American Indian Culture

However, we should return to North America to examine the use of the Candles which are but one manifestation of the important part that fire, smoke and heat plays in the diverse culture of the different Native American tribes. According to tradition everything the Creator makes has a Spirit, so everything is related and all things are sacred. There is continuity between our ancestors and those in the present and mutual respect should also extend to a respect for each other.

Also according to tradition there is a boundary between the world of the spirits and our own world and those people blessed with special characteristics and powers will be able to transcend both worlds. These people and those who wish to assume special powers often need to experience visions when the spirits and spirit powers appear. A crucial stage in experiencing visions is a ritual purification which is undergone in a sweat lodge. Other methods of receiving visions are through fasting, experiencing intense pain, exhaustion as brought about by the famous 'Ghost Dance'; communal singing and drumming and the ingestion of the spineless peyote cactus which provides a hallucinogenic drug.

Another use for smoke is for the cleansing of the body's aura by wafting a smouldering bundle of herbs, preferably sage, a few inches above and along the body.

Any fan of 'Western' films will also know that communications over long distance could be made by 'smoke signals' from one person to another.

The Hopi Tribe

As healing ear candles are associated with the Hopi tribe it may be useful to look at their way of life. The word 'Hopi' means peaceful and this epitomises their way of life. They live in adobe dwellings made from mud brick which have a roof of sticks, grass and mud supported by wooden beams. The houses were joined together to form pueblos (Spanish for 'villages') on the tops of mesa outcrops and in canyon wall recesses.

According to legend the world we now live in is the fourth way of life - different Hopi clans and animals emerged into the current way of life and when Ma'saw offered the people of the world ears of corn the Hopi were left with the smallest ears as others had pushed in before them. Together with the ear of corn the Hopi inherited their homeland, culture and responsibilities. The Hopi fulfil their responsibilities through ceremony; their way of life revolves around agriculture, especially corn. The Hopi only learn the story of their clan but this is not written down but handed down through the generations by means of drawings and verbal stories and legends.

The Hopi live mainly in the Colorado River area and the tribal farmers, hunters and gatherers would descend hundreds of feet to where they deep-planted corn. Bread was baked; wicker baskets and pots were crafted and brightly coloured cloth was made from dyed cotton cloth.

It was inevitable that the exceptional idea of ear candling and the ear candles would become known to a wider audience and so it was in the 1980s that a German company Biosun obtained the original recipe for the Candles and with modification, research and official testing produced them for a worldwide market. Their Candles can now be found in many countries and on several continents. They are not the only company producing Candles and indeed home-making Candles kits can be purchased on the internet.

Construction of Modern Ear Candles

Many people are confused about the construction of ear candles. Instead of being a traditional solid candle with a wick which is lit with the hot wax running down to the base an ear candle is usually cylindrical up to 12 inches in length with a hollow centre and no wick inside. Wax does not run down on the outside of the candle unless it is either of poor quality or being incorrectly used. The only usual visible result of the burning process is the formation of a fine ash column which may or may not separate from the candle. Ear candles can also be triangular in shape.

It is important that the end of the ear candle nearer the entrance to the ear canal is not tapered. It should not be possible to push it up the canal as this would bring it nearer to the ear drum which needs to receive maximum protection. A cylindrical shape is best as it cannot override the protective curved shape of the canal.

Most makes of ear candle come in one size so use on a person with a small entrance to the ear canal, such as a child, is best carried out by a trained, experienced therapist.

Ear candles are usually sold in pairs so that each ear can be treated during a treatment session. There is a possibility of making an ear sore if both candles are used to treat the same ear during a session. For balancing purposes, each ear should be treated during the same session.

An ear candle should contain a filter (preferably plastic), a few inches from the end of the candle, which will protect the ear canal from any wax or excessive herbal powder residue being deposited therein. The design of the filter in the original Biosun Hopi Ear Candles resembles the spiritual shape of 'mother earth' as perceived by Native American Indians.

The ear candles should be similar in length with a uniform safety marker line, drawn and positioned on the outside surface of each, below which the candle should not in any circumstance be burnt. It should be made clear on the written instructions which end of the candle is to be lit. This will ensure there is no risk of the internal filter being melted by the flame reaching it. If it is very quickly realised that the wrong end has been lit extinguish the flame and trim the burnt end - it should be possible to reuse the candle.

The best ear candles for a therapist to use have a vertical seam running from the top end of the candle to the bottom end. There will be an overlap of structure material and this will result in the candle ash leaning in a column away from the face. The cold ash column is usually black or grey; it may contain red 'beads' which are hot. Other candles which have a spiral shaped seam are not so helpful to the therapist.

The Ingredients of Ear Candles

It is important to know the ingredients of the ear candles being used to minimise any risk of an adverse reaction by the person being candled (the 'receiver'). This is an important factor to consider if ear candles containing essential oils are being used. The ingredients should be natural, organically grown if possible and the structure of the ear candle (normally cotton or linen) in which the ingredients are impregnated should not be paraffin based. The structure should be sturdy enough to keep its shape during the burning process and not melt, burn unduly or deform at any time.

The ear candles should be supplied in a transparent, hygienic sealed bag or container with information about the ingredients and clear instructions of how to use them safely. Candles originating in the European Union should always be marked with a medical devices approval CE mark and number (EEC) and there should also be a batch number. If there are any problems when using an ear candle the burning should be stopped immediately and the supplier informed within a reasonable time. A reputable shop or other outlet will always give a refund of purchase price or offer a replacement pair of ear candles upon proof of purchase. The manufacturer should be alerted to any problems by a supplier.

Ear candles normally have a long shelf life but because the treatment is so pleasant this consideration is not normally important. Candles should be kept out of warm, direct sunlight to stop them melting and deforming. They often have a pleasant fragrance and this can enhance a clothes cupboard if stored therein. If an ear candle is squashed it can often be reshaped and used.

Properties of the ingredients contained in the Ear Candles

Although any number of healing ingredients can be impregnated into the structure of an ear candle which are released by heat during the candle's burning the ingredients listed below are contained within the original Biosun candles which are used by many therapists and approved by insurance companies in the UK. qualified aromatherapists will know that each of the ingredients will have a large number of different properties.

Honey extracts
Honey and bee pollen products such as propolis have been clinically shown to have many healing properties for many conditions including helping sufferers with hay fever (allergic rhinitis). They work on the same basis as homeopathy by treating like with like. Taking a small amount regularly helps the body build resistance to invading antigens/ allergens; normally, the body releases antibodies/immunoglobulins to fight antigens. The antibodies release histamine and other chemicals which can cause swelling and irritation in the body's tissue.

Honey has been known for its healing properties for thousands of years and its early advocates include the Egyptian Pharaohs, Aristotle and Hippocrates. As well as containing sugars, honey also contains many minerals including iron, calcium and copper. The best honey for someone is either that produced in the user's neighbourhood or the Munuka honey of New Zealand.

Pure Beeswax

Beeswax is a strong antiseptic and is also anti-inflammatory.

Sage (Salvia Officinalis)

This herb is anti-inflammatory and astringent (a tightening of the skin with constriction of the blood vessels with reduced blood flow and mucous secretions together with a reduction in the ability to absorb water).Interestingly, astringent drugs are used to promote healing of broken or inflamed skin and to treat otitis externa (infection causing inflammation of the external ear canal) and watering of the eye when there is a minor irritation. Astringent drugs can cause burning or stinging when administered. Sage contains camphor so as the Biosun candles contain this herb they should not be used on epileptics as this ingredient may 'trigger' a seizure. Sage is the most revered herb used by Native American Indians and is the flower of the state of Nevada.

St John's Wort (Hypericum Perforatum)

This yellow flowered plant is anti-inflammatory and astringent. It is gently relaxing, has a restorative effect on the nervous system and in Germany is often prescribed as an antidepressant.

Chamomile (Anthemis Nobilis - Roman Chamomile)

This perennial daisy herb is anti-inflammatory, astringent and is useful for mental stress, anxiety and nervous excitability. Because it helps menstruation it should be avoided in the first three months of pregnancy (by both the client and the therapist).

Beta-Carotene/ Vitamin A

This was the first of the thirteen vitamins to be discovered. It fights infections, strengthens the immune system and is good for the skin. Carotene is present in many foods including green vegetables, tomatoes, oranges, plums, peaches and especially in carrots. Vitamin A is found in liver, egg yolk, dairy produce and margarine.

Although different essential oils such as bergamot or eucalyptus can be added to candles the therapist must ensure that the client will not have intolerance to these different ingredients. In aromatherapy a patch test is usually carried out but this safeguard is not applicable before using the candles because of their nature.

An Ear Candling therapy session

Before describing the actions of the candles and how they work it is probably useful to outline what will happen and what the 'receiver' (client/ patient) will experience during a full treatment session. To take into account the arrival of the receiver, completion of a written questionnaire, burning of candles, the face and neck massage and a recovery period approximately one hour should be allocated to a full treatment session. The treatment will be shorter if the massage, which is not obligatory, does not happen. If a treatment is carried out at an exhibition or in a GP practice less time will be spent by the therapist/ practitioner.

It should be remembered that all therapists/ practitioners are individuals and different techniques will be practised especially with the massage sequence. On the whole the following will take place;

- the receiver will be asked certain questions if a telephone enquiry about the treatment has been received especially dealing with contra-indications which will preclude against the treatment taking place e.g. is there a perforated ear drum or a grommet in place?

- when the receiver arrives for a treatment he/she is made welcome and a full written consultation takes place which will ask for certain information such as private details, medical history and any prescribed medication or medical treatment which is being carried out at the time

- the therapist will observe usual therapy professional standards of hygiene such as short fingernails and clean hands, neat hair and minimum jewellery

- the therapist should explain how the treatment will be carried out and reassure the receiver about the physical effects and results the treatment may bring about - a 'sizzling' noise and possible warmth in the ear; very rarely a blocking/unblocking feeling; drainage of nose, throat or tear duct with fluid running down the throat or nose and/ or a lightening of the head and the beginning of a headache

- the therapist should visually inspect the auricle/pinna of the ear and the skin surrounding the ear. If trained, the therapist can use an otoscope/ auriscope to check the outer ear canal for damage or blockage, inflamed skin, excessive ear wax or reflection (or lack of) of the otoscope light back from the ear drum

- the receiver should remove shoes and any heavy overclothing, loosen a tie and place any jewellery or valuables in a safe place. If he/she is worried about the massage medium staining a shirt or blouse this item of clothing can be taken off, with a towel being draped over the upper body for modesty purposes

- an asthma sufferer should be requested to bring his/her inhaler in case of a reaction (none known to the author to date)

- a hearing aid should be removed

- the receiver lies on the side on the surface of a therapy couch, normally on the side with the better ear (if there is one) uppermost. The receiver can however lie on the front or back (e.g. with a lady in the later stages of pregnancy) if this is more comfortable but it is essential that the candle is able to protrude vertically, or so, from the ear. It may be necessary to use more than one head supporting pillow and other pillows may be needed if the receiver has any medical problems, back problems in particular. Treatment can be carried out with the receiver sitting in a chair with the head tilted and supported.

- once the receiver is settled comfortable, a body covering such as a towel or blanket can be used for warmth. During many types of complementary treatment the body's temperature can drop dramatically

- treatments can be carried out on a 'relaxator' type lounger which many reflexologists use for their treatments. The receiver can even be treated in a wheelchair as long as the head can be tilted (with comfortable ear support) to allow the candle to be inserted correctly in the ear. The treatment should never be done on a bed or other moveable surface **and certainly an individual should not use the candles on him/herself**

- the therapist should be seated comfortably at a higher level than the receiver at the head of the couch with the receiver as close as possible for comfort and safety purposes. The therapist can rest the arms on a pillow which is better than a cushion for this purpose. If a therapist is short, the treatment can be done with him/her in a standing position for part or all of the session

- it may be appropriate to play relaxing music, have a sympathetic level of lighting and certainly a draught-free warm room with heating at cold times. In the summer be careful of the use of a fan as this may affect both the safety of the burning of the candle and artificially speed up the process with the full benefit of the candle's action not being experienced. Great care must be taken not to burn candles too close to sensitive smoke/heat alarms

- all equipment should be close to hand and a couch should have a cloth cover and fresh couch roll for hygiene reasons

- the therapist will cover the ear with a large protective cloth with a slit to allow entry for the candle. Between the ear and the candle there can be a tissue for additional hygiene.

An unlit candle is placed in the ear (sometimes with a twist, and a gentle pull on the ear lobe especially with a narrow entrance to the ear canal so as to obtain a good seal) so that the receiver feels what it is like. The candle is removed and lit horizontally away from the therapist, receiver and the couch, placed correctly upright in the ear and burnt down to the marker limit line. The candle is removed and directly extinguished in an adjacent bowl of water. The candle is never blown out as ash will be spread around the room, other safety steps include;

- if there is a small amount of candle residue powder at the entrance to the ear canal this is carefully wiped away using a baby bud or cloth - the bud is not pushed up into the canal itself

- the candle should be secured between the first two fingers of either hand, with the remaining fingers and the other hand resting on the receiver's head for reassurance. It is important that the pressure of the resting hand or the candle does not become uncomfortable for the receiver as the therapist relaxes into the treatment session - if the pressure becomes uncomfortable the receiver should inform the therapist who will reduce it

- it is important that the correct end of the candle is lit and that if the candle has a straight seam this should point towards the receiver's nose. As the treatment should be carried out in a draught free room the ash will fall away from the face. If the ash, which is not usually hot, falls toward the face this is an indication that the candle has not been seated in the entrance to the ear canal in the right position. If smoke is seen coming from the base of the candle it has to repositioned, not removed, at a different angle or deeper to stop this happening.

During each treatment the following will happen;

- the receiver turns on to the second, sometimes the worst side and the procedure of the first ear repeated; if a lighter is used it should be on a low flame setting

- the therapist will note the burning time of each candle on a treatment record card for comparative purposes. The difference in times is an indicator of the state of the ears and surrounding facial structures

- the face and neck massage sequence will then take place with the receiver on his/her back with eyes closed to avoid any accidents. The massage can be done with or without massage medium such as oil or cream; the skin normally has enough moisture to allow the therapist's fingers to slide over the skin. It is important that the therapist checks that the receiver has no intolerance to the ingredients to be used. The massage enhances the actions of the candles and has specific healing purposes which should be explained to the receiver beforehand. If the receiver does not want a massage his/ her wishes should be respected

- it is likely that a client's hairstyle will be ruffled by the massage no matter how careful the therapist is (a hair band can be used). It is important to know whether the recipient is wearing contact lenses (which do not have to be removed) as their presence may necessitate different massage moves being carried out

- the massage sequence and individual moves should be tailored to the needs of the recipient e.g. if the sinuses need draining, specific sinus drainage points should be activated; if the neck's muscles are tense this area should be concentrated on

- the therapist should be aware of the pressure being used during the insertion of the candles and the massage and this pressure should be comfortable for the receiver. At all times the receiver has the right to ask for modifications to the massage if they are safe and practicable, **and also to ask for either part of the treatment (candling and massage) to be stopped if undue discomfort or any pain is experienced**

- after the completion of the massage the receiver should rest for a while, slowly get up and have a drink of water. The therapist will explain the significance of the remnants inside the candles when they have been opened and other indicators which arose during the treatment such as the length of burning and any smoke which may have been seen. Short and long term advice will be given and the date for the next treatment recommended

- the receiver will gather together belongings, replace shoes and over clothing and, after paying the therapist's fee, leave; the therapist will have a drink of water, write up any notes and the treatment record card, which can be used for comparative purposes next time, and await the next client.

A Suggested List of items needed for a Treatment Session

The following equipment is needed to carry out a treatment;
1. consultation form
2. treatment record card
3. pen or pencil
4. firm therapist's couch (or similar)
5. comfortable therapist's stool/chair - shorter therapists can stand
6. couch cover and couch roll
7. pillow(s) to support the receiver's head and body
8. blanket(s) - especially to cover the receiver's feet
9. pair of ear candles
10. matches/lighter
11. dish of water in which to extinguish the candles

12.   protective towel or cloth, with a hole, to be placed over the receiver's ear
13.   tissues
14.   cotton baby buds
15.   massage oil or cream
16.   clock or watch
17.   side trolley
18.   waste paper bin
19.   suitable relaxing music
20.   receptacle for the receiver's jewellery or valuables
21.   drinks of water for the receiver and therapist at the end of the session.

How Do The Ear Candles Work?

Like many therapists, I was often puzzled by fundamental questions including;
● How do the candles work?
● Why do candles take different lengths of time to burn with different people and in the opposite ears of the same person?
● What were the often disgusting looking remnants lying above the candle filter which were revealed when the cooled burnt candle was opened and what did they signify?
● Why do some candles smoke when they are being burnt and others do not?
● What is the 'sizzling' noise heard by receivers during candle burning?

I must confess that I have altered my views about the therapy over time with the great number of treatments I have supervised and carried out since my own training in 1997. The greatest shift in my views however has been precipitated by the use of the otoscope to check the condition of the ear canals before I begin the treatment. This is a wonderful aid to any 'Ear candler' in his/her work; it is advisable however that they receive instruction in its use and that a disposable speculum is used for each ear unless access can be gained to the correct sterilisation equipment.

Laboratory comparison and analysis of unused and used candles

In January 2004 the author (at great expense) commissioned the accredited Reading Scientific Services laboratory to test the Biosun Original Hopi Ear Candles by comparing and analysing a new, unburnt pair of candles and the remains of four pairs of candles which had been burnt within one hour of each other. The new and burnt candles were from the same batch.

The burnt candles contained residues of yellowish powder and wax. These residues were examined by light microscopy, photographed and analysed by Fourier infrared (FT-IR) spectroscopy and x-ray microanalysis. The residues (both powdery material and waxy material) were found to be composed predominantly of beeswax. No ear wax, skin cells or hairs were detected. FT-IR analysis of wax isolated from an unused candle produced a similar spectrum to that of the residues.

10

This test confirms what the author had thought in that the residue wax in the candles was from the candles (beeswax) and is not ear wax. A simple experiment to reinforce this view is by burning a candle down to a marker line (if there is one), allowing it to cool and then opening it. The result should be some wax and powder. Furthermore, the author examined a pair of ears which did not have any visible ear wax through an otoscope before a treatment; after burning, the candles when opened contained a great deal of wax - which could not have come from the ears. The ears belonged to an elderly lady with severe hearing problems. These burnt candles are used as a teaching tool during the author's accredited courses.

The Physical and Aromatherapy Actions of the Ear Candles

I hope that the information I give below will fit into the pattern of the vast majority of treatments which are carried out by therapists. On my own courses I always open the candles I have used on my volunteer during my practical demonstration with some nervousness but in virtually all the cases what I have told my students before the opening event has proved to be correct. Having taught over 1,600 students I have used up a lot of nervous energy to date (November 2005)!

The Physical Actions

Once the therapist and receiver are comfortable, a candle is lit and placed correctly upright in the entrance to the ear canal with the protective cloth in place. After a short while the herbs, wax and honey ingredients (or similar) which are impregnated in the cotton or linen structure are vaporised and drawn down inside the hollow inside of the candle. The sizzling sound which is heard by the receiver is that of the ingredients vaporising at different rates. It is at this time that, depending on the state of the ear and head environment, some of the herbs are turned to a fine yellow powder and some of the wax solidifies. Crucially, for safety purposes, all the wax and nearly all the herbal powder residue (which is cool) remain above the candle's integral protective polyethylene (PE) plastic filter (or similar) if there is one.

According to the manufacturers of the Biosun Traditional Hopi Ear Candles - who seem to be the only candles manufacturers to have carried out any research - 'a light suction action (the chimney effect) occurs and the movement of the candle flame creates a vibration of herbal vapour which generates a massaging effect on the ear drum and also the ossicle bones which are linked to its posterior part. This action mimics that of sound (pressure) waves which are also transmitted down the ear canal to the ear drum. The oxygen in the ear canal is replaced by the vapours which begin to move in a current through the filter with the down draught on the left and right side of the hollow centre with the up draught in the middle of the centre of the candle'. As the receiver can hear the sizzling noise caused by the action of the candle this indicates that there is no vacuum as sound has to be transmitted across a solid material, gas or fluid and this is not possible when a vacuum has been created.

It is essential to facilitate the gentle movement of the vapours by ensuring that the candle is seated tightly at the entrance to the ear canal so that a seal is made and no vapour smoke can escape at this point. If vapours escape simply adjust the depth or angle of the candle. No vapour will pass through an intact ear drum into the middle ear.

The temperature increase in the ear canal is then transmitted through to the rest of the ear and the surrounding structures such as the nose and sinuses. The change in temperature will lead to a change in pressure and an expansion in these areas, which have often become congested with conditions such as sinusitis or rhinitis, which hopefully will lead to them draining and clearing. It is this reaction which receivers often experience when they are having their ears 'candled' and which leads to fluid trickling down the throat. According to Charles law of physics 'The volume of a given mass of gas at constant pressure is directly proportionate to its absolute temperature'.

The circulation of vapours is very gentle and their temperature and strength is such that it is not possible to remove any wax which may be contained within the ear canal. Any minute black specks which are visible in the wax within the candles when they are opened are probably dirt or dust which has accumulated near the canal entrance and which are the result of work or leisure activities such as building work or decorating.

Because some ear wax/cerumen, if it is present in any great amount, is warmed, moistened and loosened by the warmth of the candles this may lead to a minute amount falling out over the next 48 hours either by the force of gravity or after a warm shower, sauna, session on the beach or similar activity when the ear is externally warmed. This movement of wax may in fact lead to a diminution of hearing which can be a similar experience for someone using ear drops which may hydrate and expand ear wax.

The circulation of the herbally enriched vapours within the outer ear canal which leads to the entire ear and surrounding structures being warmed with changes in pressure when combined and reinforced by the face and neck massage will form an overall holistic treatment. When taken together they will;
● sooth irritated areas (ingredients)
● stimulate peripheral blood circulation (massage and heat)
● strengthen the immune system (ingredients)
● strengthen the work of the lymphatic system (massage and heat)
● stimulate energy points on the external ear (position of the candle, heat and massage)

The Aromatherapy Actions

As we have seen, ear candles are made up of natural ingredients which have accepted healing and soothing properties. The receiver will benefit from the action of the warmed herbal vapours which act physically within the body and also from the inhalation of the fragrance of the different vapours in their entirety.

Vapours are initially detected in the nasal mucosa, which contain millions of olfactory receptor cells. Odour molecules are warmed and filtered with attendant stimulation of olfactory neurones (nerve cells).

It can be said that the physiological and psychological benefits of the inhalation of the fragrance is demonstrated by the promotion of relaxation and stress reduction (the 'Cephalic' effects) which leads to both a promotion of a positive mental state and also a likelihood of reducing blood pressure and associated conditions such as strokes and heart disease. The stimulation of the olfactory system is transferred to the limbic part of the brain which has association with memory, emotions and 'feeling good'.

There will also be an enhancement of the body's immune system. Molecules enter the respiratory system and attach themselves to oxygen molecules in the lungs which are then transported around the body to the various organs, tissues and cells. The result is that the body can defend itself better against infections.

Because of the proximity of the therapist to the vapours, he/ she will also derive the same benefits, but to a lesser extent, as the receiver from this major part of the overall treatment. The author has often found that after a day's teaching of this therapy, which includes observing up to thirteen treatments that some debris is loosened from his own ears, the lungs feel clearer, as do the sinuses.

Results of the Burning of the Ear Candles

The different results of the ear candling are due to the condition of the ears and surrounding structures and not from the candles themselves. Many people think that the action of the candles will depend on the state of the ear canal and how it is affected by its shape, excessive wax, dirt, age of receiver and so on. Obviously these are factors, but we should consider the ear (and its outer canal) as part of the inner head. Conditions and any problems which arise should be considered in the wider context of the head as a whole.

There are several pointers which should be taken into account when assessing the result of the treatment and thus when the receiver should be recommended by the therapist to return for the next treatment. **Because many conditions are chronic/ long standing it is recommended that three sessions should comprise an initial course of treatment.** The intervals between these sessions being dependant mainly on what is found in the filters after the candles have been opened and how the receiver's health has reacted to the treatment. These intervals are guidelines and the receiver can come within a shorter interval if the therapy is being enjoyed and is proving beneficial or if environmental reasons cause a change in head health. If after three sessions nothing positive is being gained, the therapist should offer the receiver advice about alternative options which are available.

There are five indicators which help the therapist to determine what is happening and to advise on the interval before the next treatment;

- the length of time each candle takes to burn down to the limit indicator line
- whether, and the amount and colour of, candle smoke during the burning
- the level of the 'sizzling' sound heard during the burning
- the appearance and amount of debris in the candles after they are opened
- how the receiver feels after the treatment and between treatments.

The length of time for the Candle to burn

It is important that the candles should be burnt in a draught free room to minimise the possibility of artificially speeding up the process. If one candle takes longer to burn than the other then this is probably the receiver's worst side. It is also useful to compare burning times during different sessions; hopefully the time of the second and subsequent sessions will be less as the head problem and condition should be improved by the treatments.

The amount and colour of the Candle smoke

Most receivers look forward to being told that a large amount of smoke has been produced by the candles during their session and that this is an indication that the ears have been cleaned. In reality, it is only a tiny percentage of ears which produce smoke. It has also been observed that the smoke can be produced when candles are used in ears which have little or no wax and often in these cases when the smoke is being produced wax can remain in the candles when they are opened up at the end of a session. Some smoke is little in amount and intermittently produced whilst other amounts of smoke can be voluminous and constant during the burning. Sometimes smoke will emit from one candle and not the other.

I would suggest the following answers to these conundrums;

- if smoke is seen in any large amount, this will indicate that the receiver may have a problem(s) with the head environment, very rarely will the candle filter be completely clear after a large amount of smoke has been emitted
- smoke will emit from the side of the head which is affected more by diverse conditions such as impaired hearing, blocked ear canal, sinusitis, hay fever, migraines, TMJ problems, neck problems etc
- If smoke comes from both sides; the greater the amount from one side indicates that the problem is worse on that side
- the darker the colour of the smoke - the worse is the condition(s)
- if no smoke is emitted; it is likely that the receiver is quite healthy with few ENT problems.

The 'Sizzling' Sound heard by the receiver during the Candle burning

The 'sizzling' sound which is heard by most receivers, and is likened to bacon frying in a pan, while the candle is burning is caused by the burning and vaporising of the herbal, honey and beeswax ingredients which are impregnated within a candle's cotton or linen structure. It is probable that the ingredients do not burn and vaporise at a constant speed (and some may be unburnt) so this is why the sound is not constant.

The sound should increase as the flame advances towards the limit line as this is physically nearer the ear drum. The sound should be more perceptible in an ear which has its outer ear canal clearer than the other ear canal. The sound should also be more perceptible in the ear which has the better overall hearing and is not so affected by conductive or sensorineural hearing loss caused by whatever means.

In rare cases the receiver will experience a 'popping' or 'blocking'/'unblocking' sensation; this is similar to that felt in the ears when flying. This process is most likely to be the result of the action of the opening of the Eustachian tube which has been affected by the warmth from the candle rather than a warming/ softening of the wax within the ear canal.

The appearance and meaning of the debris in an opened Candle after it has been burned

Probably the most interesting, and informative part of the whole treatment for both therapist and receiver is when the candles are opened after they have been allowed to cool (possibly while the massage is being carried out) and any material remaining allowed to harden. The results are the most important determinant of when the recipient should return for the next treatment.

Often, the result in one ear will be different to the result in the other ear. This is another indicator for the therapist to gain confirmation of the inner head health of the recipient. The aim of the treatments is to progress from one result to a better result; mainly because of environmental factors and susceptibility to allergens, infections and flu, it is unlikely that the candles become completely clear.

These are the following possible results which are brought about by the action of the candles together with the condition of the 'head environment' of the recipient;

1.   The best result - nothing visible/remaining in the candle
2.   The next best result - yellow powder (candle herbal residue) visible
3.   The nearly worst result - wax (beeswax which is from the candle and not ear wax) visible
4.   The worst result - yellow powder and wax visible.

1. Nothing remaining in the candle

This is a very unusual result and the few people in this situation have mainly been ladies from the Indian sub continent culture who have good head health and a history of family care in ear cleaning, usually using oils, from an early age.

The process that leads to the good result happening is that the candle's heat energy vapours circulate within the ear canal. Because there are no problems in the ear canal other parts of the ear and adjacent structures the candles do not have to lose any energy trying to deal with a problem/ condition. No heat is lost around the ear drum and all the ascending smoke energy is available to burn off the honey, herbs and wax which are coming down the inside of the candle. Usually the burning time of a candle in a 'good' ear is approximately 9.5 - 10 minutes. If the time is less than this, the positioning of the candle in the ear and any draughts in the room should be checked.

2. Yellow powder remaining in the Candle

The powder remaining in the candle is the same colour as the candle and this gives a clue to its ingredients - which are the herbs impregnated within the cotton structure. Most people whose candles only have yellow powder are on the whole 'head healthy'. The ear with a greater amount of powder remaining is the worse of the two ears. The burning process which leads to just yellow powder remaining is the same as when there is nothing remaining i.e. there is heat energy circulating within the ear canal.

In this case, the recipient may be suffering mildly from condition(s) such as rhinitis, sinusitis or a light cold. The candle senses this situation and tries to treat the condition(s) accordingly. Some of the heat energy is lost around the ear drum and not so much is rising to burn off all the vaporised ingredients which are descending the inside of the candle. There is still enough available to burn off the wax but not the herbs and it is these in powder form which remain either in a single column or in small pieces.

Sometimes, a little of the herbal residue powder, which is cool, may descend past the plastic filter and lie at the entrance to the ear canal. The powder residue can be wiped away by the therapist. If a cylindrical shaped candle is used there is little risk of the powder migrating up the ear canal because of the canal's shape. If any powder is missed by the therapist it will be removed during the massage or by gravity or by the ear's natural self-cleansing action over the next few days after the treatment.

Usually, the burning time of a candle with yellow powder will be approximately 10 - 10.5 minutes. If one candle has more powder than the other then this has probably been inserted in the side with more problems and consequently it will take longer to burn.

3. Wax remaining in the Candle

The dull red colour of the wax which is found in the Candle after burning is not the same as the colour of wax which is seen in the ear canal with an otoscope/auriscope which can range from yellow through bright red to brown or even black (impacted ear wax on the ear drum). Although the circulating vapour has energy this is not enough to raise ear wax up one inch, from where it is seated at the entrance to the canal, through the plastic filter and above the filter. The only items which could be removed by the vapours are specks of dirt or dust which were in the canal near to its entrance. The burning process is the same as that which gave the first two results - heat energy from the vaporised ingredients circulating within the ear canal.

In this case, the recipient is suffering more seriously from a condition(s) such as flu, headache or severe sinusitis. The candle senses the worse condition and has to work harder to try to treat it. Consequently, more energy is used up around the ear drum and even less remains available to burn off the ingredients which are migrating down the inside of the candle. Enough ascending heat is available to burn off the descending herbal powder but there is not enough to burn off the wax. The worse the condition, the more energy is lost so more wax will remain. The wax can either be seen in a long 'string' or as small particles in different parts of the remainder of the candle above the filter.

The presence of an efficient filter, which should be situated well above the bottom end of the candle, is essential to minimise the risk of any hot wax entering and damaging the ear canal or ear drum.

Usually, the burning time of a candle with wax remaining will be approximately 10.5 - 11 minutes and the candle containing more beeswax and which takes longer to burn will have been inserted in the ear on the side of the head with the worse problem(s).

4. Yellow Powder and Beeswax remaining in the Candle

The burning process which gives the result of yellow powder and wax in the candle is the same as in the first three results mentioned above - heat energy from the vaporised ingredients circulating within the ear canal.

In this case, the recipient is suffering badly from an acute or chronic (or both) condition which may be causing misery or pain (or both) such as a migraine, painful teeth, flu and neuralgia. The candle detects and tries to address the seriousness of the problem and consequently most of its energy is dissipated around the ear drum. A minimal amount remains to burn off the descending herbs, honey and wax and the result is that most of them will remain in the candle as powder and wax appearing as a whole column or broken up into pieces. Again, the filter will prevent any of the wax passing into the ear canal.

Usually, the burning time of a candle with powder and wax will be in excess of 11 minutes and the candle containing more powder and wax and which takes longer to burn will have been inserted in the ear on the side of the head with the worse problem(s).

How the receiver feels after, and between, treatments

Probably the most important measure of the success of any treatment - medical or complementary, is how the patient/receiver feels after it. This is as true with ear candling as any other treatment.**The effects of the candling will continue for up to 48 hours and within this period it is not necessary to have a subsequent treatment. If the treatment is done within this time there is a possibility of making the ears sore.**

Very often there will be an instantaneous improvement of a problem; the nasal area or sinuses may start to drain with the head feeling lighter. Whilst this can happen, often the recipient will initially feel nothing and in fact occasionally the symptoms can get worse. A worsening situation is called a 'healing process' and the therapist should inform the recipient that this may occur. The 48 hour after-treatment period is important and many who develop a headache on the way home will feel better the next morning.

When a receiver returns for a subsequent treatment the therapist should always refer to case notes and enquire what has happened in the intervening period since the previous session with special regard to specific ENT conditions and the general health situation. If progress is being made and the second treatment seems promising then both parties can become confident of the outcome.

Unfortunately, one of the modern trends in life is to expect instant solutions. This is true with regard to treatments for mind, body and spirit problems. The candling therapy should not be judged on one result alone even though this may have been successful. **Three treatments is an initial course and if improvements are being experienced further treatments should be considered. If improvements are not happening then the therapist should offer additional options and advice.**

Ranking of treatment indicators

The therapist has several indicators which occur during a treatment to influence his/ her thoughts on the success of the therapy and when the next treatment should be scheduled. I would consider that these should be ranked as follows;
1. **how the receiver feels after experiencing the treatment and between treatments**
2. **what the remnants in the candles suggest regarding the interval before the next treatment**
3. **the length of time of burning each candle**
4. **whether and how each candle smokes**
5. **the level of the 'sizzling' sound which is perceived by the receiver.**

Interval of time between treatments

It is recommended that three or four sessions constitute an initial course of treatments especially if the condition(s) has been chronic for a long period. The candles both treat the condition and are also a preventative. Their ingredients should strengthen the body's immune system which will help the body's defences to act against incoming harmful viruses and allergens.

It is suggested that 48 hours elapse between treatments to allow the candles' actions to work and to minimise the risk of making the ears sore. Although the following intervals are guidelines it is up to each therapist to take each case on its individual merits. If the recipient is either benefiting from the treatment or unexpectedly suffers from an ENT problem there is no reason why he/ she cannot come sooner than the periods recommended;

1. **Nothing visible in the candles:**   **2 months before the next treatment**
2. **Yellow powder in either candle:**   **1-2 months before the next treatment**
3. **Wax in either candle:**   **7 days-1 month before the next treatment**
4. **Wax and powder in either candle:**   **2-7 days before the next treatment.**

If one candle has one result and the other has a worse result the interval should be connected to the worse candle e.g. one candle = wax; the other = powder, the interval is recommended to be 7 days - 1 month i.e. the interval for wax presence.

Position of the therapist

Most professional treatments will be carried out with a seated therapist and the client lying on a suitable firm couch. It is recommended that the therapist sits comfortably, with arms supported by a wide pillow(s) or towel, at the head of the couch with the client's head as close as possible to the therapist and all equipment nearby. The advantages of sitting at the head, and not the side, of the couch are;

● the therapist does not lean across the client's body and aura
● the therapist can protect the client's shoulder from the candle's flame better if the client's shoulder relaxes and moves
● the therapist can keep in contact with the client continuously
● Reiki or other healing can be given easily because the therapist's hands are placed on the client's head
● if there are time constraints, such as during an exhibition, the therapist can do the face and neck massage at the same time as the candle is burning.

Contraindications against the use of the Ear Candles Therapy

It is important for a therapist to consider whether there are any circumstances or conditions which will preclude using the candling therapy on a prospective receiver or when the receiver returns for a subsequent treatment. This philosophy also hold true for other complementary therapies and conventional medical treatments.

As the therapy consists of the application/ burning of a pair of ear candles and the face/ neck massage both of these aspects should be considered. It would be useful to explain what the treatment consists of and also the contraindications when receiving an initial telephone, written or personal enquiry as this may save embarrassment for either party when the prospective receiver arrives the first time for a treatment. The therapist can only be guided by, and act accordingly on, the information given by the receiver. The verbal questioning and written consultation form, which should be signed by the receiver, are most important.

Contraindications against the use of the Candles
1.   If the ear drum is perforated, or if a perforation has healed in the last 3 months (a healing process)
2.   If a grommet, or other drainage device, is in place in the ear drum or has fallen out in the past 3 months
3.   if the receiver is allergic to any of the candle's ingredients - if honey is an ingredient, this will not directly enter the digestive system; St Johns Wort in this form is unlikely to act against a long term antidepressant drug such as Prozac
4.   if the receiver is under specific medical supervision
5.   if a course of antibiotics or other short term medication is being followed for ENT condition(s) - wait until this medication has been completed
6.   if severe dental work, such as root canal fillings or the removal of wisdom teeth, has left the jaw and face sore and possibly in spasm
7.   if a current 'healing process' is underway
8.   if the receiver is unable to tilt the head so that the candles cannot be inserted in an (almost) upright position
9.   if a lady is in the first trimester (first 12 weeks) of pregnancy - if sage (a stimulant) is one of the candle's ingredients - this contraindication also applies to the therapist
10. if the surroundings or equipment being used are not safe - there may be draughts or the treatment couch is wobbly
11. if no responsible adult is available to be present when a minor (under 16 years of age) is being treated. This proviso applies to all therapies
12. if the receiver has epilepsy - the ingredient sage contains camphor which rarely may precipitate a seizure
13. if the receiver has a fever or an infectious condition - this also applies to the therapist
14. if a cochlear implant is fitted or if a hearing aid is in position
15. if a mastoidectomy operation has taken place
16. a child under 3 years of age - because the ear entrance will be small
17. it is unlikely that the candles will affect the action of contraceptive pills containing oestrogen.

If the outer ear canal is inflamed due to a condition such as psoriasis or eczema being active then it is likely that the receiver will not like the candle pressing on the skin. If the condition is not present in one ear treat that ear first.

A receiver with high or low blood pressure can usually have a treatment but care has to be exercised when he/she arises from the couch to make sure the movement is not done quickly with consequent light-headedness. It is advisable that all receivers have a light meal some time before the treatment. If this has not happened a banana can be offered by the therapist to raise the receiver's blood sugar level. **If in any doubt the receiver can be asked to check with the appropriate medical practitioner before undergoing a course of treatments**

It is often a prudent idea to ask if the receiver wants to use the toilet before the treatment especially if he/she is stressed or has been on a long journey before the treatment.

Contraindications against the accompanying face and neck massage

A therapist should consider whether there are any of the usual contraindications to massage and these include;
- **fractures of bones,**
- **cuts to the skin**
- **fever or an infectious condition**
- **any pain or unexplained swelling**
- **any contagious skin condition - gloves can be worn by the therapist.**

If any massage medium (oil, cream, gel or powder) is to be used, the therapist should inform the receiver of its ingredients; if there is any risk a different, or no, medium should be used. Normally the skin contains enough moisture to allow a massage to be carried out satisfactorily.

It is advisable that only a qualified aromatherapist uses a mixture of carrier and essential oils as the massage medium or if the candles contain essential oils.

If there is any doubt whether to carry out a massage (remember, it is not mandatory) or the burning of the candles - Don't do it.

If a therapist has any doubts whether the therapy should be carried out the receiver can be referred back to a qualified medical practitioner for clarification. If a client is referred by a GP to a therapist for this or any other complementary therapy it is only sensible and good etiquette to keep the practitioner informed of the progress of the treatment.

Can anyone be treated with the Candles?

Whilst the ear candles can be used on anyone approximately over the age of three it is important that they are able to lie still during the duration of a treatment which in the case of children may only be for the length of time the candles take to burn. There is no upper age limit but an important factor is whether the receiver is able to incline the head so that the candles can be inserted in an upright position. It may be more difficult to position the correct end of a candle into the entrance of the outer ear canal of people, especially children, who have a small entrance. In this case the gentle pull on the ear lobe and the twist of the candle to get a good seal is important. In these cases the therapist has to do his/ her best. It is not advisable to shave the end of the candle to fit into the ear canal as it may be projected nearer the ear drum if done incorrectly. Even for children the candle is burnt down to the red marker line (if there is one).

Obviously all the contraindications which are listed elsewhere in this chapter must be adhered to before carrying out the treatment.

Conditions for which the Candles therapy may be useful

As we will see in Chapters 5 and 8 there are a large number of diverse ENT conditions which can lead to other conditions such as snoring and sleep apnoea. Tightness in the neck muscles and disturbance to the blood and lymphatic circulatory systems can in turn affect the ear, nose and throat and related structures.

The aim of the burning of the candles when augmented by the face and massage is to try to address many of these conditions. If the therapy is not successful then it is the function and responsibility of a good trained therapist to offer advice and other options and this is dealt with later in this chapter and in subsequent chapters.

The therapy (ear candling and massage) aims to help the following conditions (in no order of importance) in the following ways;

Snoring: Three of the factors which may lead to snoring are congestion of the upper respiratory airway; being overweight; and the loss of muscle tone and the development of fatty deposits around the throat. If the candles help with drainage of the nasal passages the necessity of needing to open the mouth to take in air with consequent vibration of the soft palate should be reduced. The therapist will also be able to give advice on having a good lifestyle including diet and exercise

Labyrinthitis: An inflammation of the balance part of the labyrinth (inner ear) caused by a viral or bacterial infection. The symptoms are vertigo and possible nausea, hearing loss and tinnitus. The warmth indirectly from the candles may help combat the infection

Sleep Apnoea: This is a problem whereby the sufferer is not able to breathe periodically for a few seconds; the drop in carbon dioxide levels is recognised by the brain and breathing is naturally restarted. Normally, an artificial airway is used to minimise the risks of this condition. If the candles are used they may be able to improve the breathing situation

Regulation of the sinuses and/ or nose: The warming action of the candles when combined with massage of specific release points should help change pressure and drain the facial sinuses and nose and reduce sinusitis and allergic rhinitis (hay fever)

Excessive or compacted ear wax (cerumen): All ears produce wax as a protective mechanism. If there is an excess or it becomes impacted on the ear drum the normal treatments are ceruminolytic drops, ear irrigation or minor surgical procedures. The wax will be warmed by the candles and may be loosened for ejection within 48 hours. One of the two natural ways that wax is moved up the ear canal is by the action of the TMJ (jaw joint) and if this is massaged it should help its efficiency

'Glue ear' (Otitis media with effusion): This form of middle ear infection which is due initially to inefficient action of the Eustachian Tube (E.T.) is more prevalent in children than adults because their E.T. is shorter and straighter and thus more prone to infection. The condition is usually treated by inserting a grommet in the ear drum through which the infection drains into the outer ear canal. Often grommet insertion has to be repeated and this may scar the ear drum. The warmth from the candle should encourage the muscular action of the E.T to work better with an improvement in opening, closing and draining. The introduction of the candle's herbal ingredients should strengthen the immune system and help fight infections.

Patulous Eustachian Tube (PET): This is a condition where the Eustachian Tube is abnormally open. The result is that the sufferer experiences all the sounds which are within the head - chewing, yawning and swallowing as well as experiencing the voice's sound which is transmitted around the bones of the skull and those sounds which are experienced by the normal mechanism of hearing. It leads to a very uncomfortable sensation and is socially inhibiting. The candle's heat should help to improve the action of the muscles surrounding the Eustachian Tube

Colds and influenza (flu): The candles can help relieve the symptoms of a cold or flu by helping to clear the airways and also by raising the level of the immune system which is responsible for fighting an allergen such as a cold virus

Headaches and migraines: The candles, and the massage, can help the blood circulation and this may reduce pressure on the nerves within the outer skull. The massage can reduce stress and neck tension which are two of the causes of headaches and migraines. Many people who suffer from migraines also have a dysfunction of the TMJ (jaw joint), the candle's warmth and the massage should improve its action

Tinnitus and other noises in the ears: Noises in the ear can have many causes. From an insect or water lodged in the outer ear canal, to disturbance of the blood supply in the upper mouth to tinnitus. Tinnitus is a complex problem, with many causes, usually within either the cochlea part of the inner ear or the acoustic nerve from the ear to the brain. While the candles may be able to dry the ear or even kill an insect its best result on tinnitus may be to reduce the noise for a short time. Their warmth may improve blood circulation in the whole ear. The massage should reduce stress levels and this may be important because stress is one of the causes of tinnitus

Ménière's Disease: This is a serious progressive inner ear problem which may be unilateral or bilateral. Its symptoms can be loss of hearing, tinnitus, vertigo, 'fullness' of the ear, 'drop' or 'shove' attacks, sickness or any combination of these. This is a complicated condition and the candles treatment may help reduce the stress of a sufferer. A therapist's after- care advice is important; such as considering joining the Ménière's Society and reducing salt intake because of its effects on the inner ear fluids

Relaxation of excessive excitement and stress: Both adults and young people can suffer with stress and hyperactivity with negative effects on their health, school work, social and economic welfare. Often people fall asleep during the burning of the candles or during the massage (or both). Relaxation can be heightened by using essential oils during the massage (if appropriate). The increase in relaxation often carries over into improved sleep patterns. If hyperactive children, especially those suffering with an attention disorder, can see colourful leaflets about the origin of the candles and observe a parent or older brother/ sister undergoing the treatment first they are more likely to be confident to try the treatment. There should always be a responsible adult present during the treatment of someone under 16 years of age

Neuralgia of a Facial Nerve: This is a pain caused by an irritation of damage to a nerve, most commonly the Facial or Trigeminal cranial nerves. If the nerve is being impinged by a blood vessel then an improvement in the circulation or nerve end relaxation by the use of the candles or the massage of the area affected may be beneficial. The occipital nerve can be irritated and this may be helped with the massage. The possible improvement of the TMJ may help swallowing and talking which have a bearing on certain neuralgias

Down's syndrome: Many people with this condition have small outer ear canals and this may the cause of ear infections and over production of wax. The candle's warmth may address these problems and stress relief may help irregular sleep patterns. A responsible person should always be present when an ear candling treatment is carried out

Bell's palsy: The symptoms of this condition, where one side of the face droops and the eye on that side is affected, can be helped by the massage and by the action of the candles on trying to keep the tear duct clear (probably not in initial stages of BP)

Blocked tear duct: If a tear duct, which drains into the nose, is blocked the candle's warmth may be able to change pressure and help clear and stimulate it

Loss or reduction of smell: The aromatherapy effects of the candle's actions help to stimulate the olfactory/ smell system; hopefully any loss of sense of smell will be recovered

'Swimmer's' or 'Surfer's Ear': These are common names for the infection Otitis externa which occurs in the outer ear canal. The astringent action of the candle's ingredients can reduce the flow of secretions. The herbal vapours will also sooth the outer ear canal and dry any infected water lodged in the ear canal

Flying or diving pressure problems: There are a number of specialities in aviation and diving medicine including conditions brought about by the ear's adverse reaction to a change in atmospheric pressure. The candle's warmth may be able to help the Eustachian Tube (whose main function is to equalise pressure in the middle ear) open and close properly and reduce pain or discomfort when airline cabin pressure is changed, especially on landing; or ascent is being made during deep sea or sub aqua diving. Diving at depth should not be considered if someone has either an ear infection or a cold so the use of the candles may help improve these conditions

Motion sickness: This is caused by the effects of repetitive movements in the inner ear balance mechanism. It can be exacerbated by worrying about the effects of previous attacks. The candles can help keep the inner ear in balance. The massage should help to reduce stress levels

Vertigo and dizziness: These symptoms are usually the result of problems with the inner ear balance mechanism and the blood supply to the brain. Dizziness can be caused by less serious triggers such as tiredness, stress and lack of food, the therapist can offer advice on these matters. Massage and the candling can help reduce stress and the workings of the inner ear environment

TMJ (Jaw joint) dysfunction: The good action of the Temporomandibular Joint (TMJ) is important as being one of the methods by which ear wax is moved away from the ear drum. TMJ problems are often experienced by migraine sufferers and it can lead to symptoms such as grinding of teeth and mouth 'clicking' noises. The candle's warmth sometimes causes the joint to become mobile; the massage can also enhance this action

Disturbance of the lymphatic system: The state of the lymph nodes and glands reflect the condition of the body in that area. If there is disease or inflammation the nearby lymph nodes will become tender and swollen. The candle's warmth and the massage should assist the Mandibular, Occipital and Cervical lymph nodes and the Parotid lymph glands in particular (see diagram opposite page 39).

Tense neck muscles: The massage should ease the neck muscles and not only should this be relaxing for the receiver but it might also reduce the onset of headaches or migraines if they are tension related.

A MASSAGE ROUTINE

A massage sequence to the face and neck follows the application of the ear candles and this holistically completes the treatment. The massage does not have to be applied;
● if there are contraindications against the massage
● if there are time constraints
● if the client does not wish to receive a massage.

If there are time constraints the massage can be done at the same time as the burning of the ear candles.

It is possible for the massage to begin the overall treatment but if the candle burning is prior to the massage these are the following advantages;
● the action of the massage will enhance the therapeutic and relaxing actions of the candles
● after a massage a client may not like to be asked to change position and lie on the side to allow the candles to be inserted and burnt in the ear
● there is no need for the therapist to wash hands after handling the candles prior to the massage- this is not the case if massage cream is used first
● the massage may expel any herbal powder residue which has been missed by the cotton bud cleansing of the entrance to the outer ear canal
● while the massage is being carried out, the remnants in the candles have time to harden prior to examination by the therapist
● there is no risk that too much time will be spent on the face and neck massage to the detriment of the time spent on the candle burning.

A client should be advised that a face and neck massage using massage cream or oil is part of the overall treatment and having been so advised a client may not wish to apply makeup or skin products before the treatment. The massage can be done without oil or cream. The massage may dishevel a hairstyle (a hair band can be used).

Aims of the massage

The neck and face massage, which follows the application of the candles, has many aims including;
● holistically completing the treatment
● enhancing the actions of the candles

- improving the blood and lymph circulation
- eliminating toxins
- helping drain the sinuses
- relaxing and destressing the client
- helping improve TMJ efficiency
- toning and relaxing muscles
- aiding skin cell desquamation/ exfoliation
- lubricating and toning the skin
- helping the therapist learn of problem areas of the face and neck which the client may have not mentioned
- stimulating auriculotherapy energy points of the ear and facial acupressure points
- opening the 'third eye' chakra point.

Massage Safety Considerations

1. Check with the client/ receiver that he/she has no allergies or intolerance to the ingredients of the massage medium (if oil, cream or talc is being used).

2. The therapist should have short, smooth fingernails and clean hands.

3. Check with the client that the pressure being used is comfortable; sometimes it may have to be increased; sometimes lessened. To enhance the benefits of the massage jewellery and spectacles should be removed if possible and ties or collar buttons loosened. Client's hair may be tied back if preferred by the client.

4. A client should always be asked if contact lenses are being worn, if this is the case then the face massage (no. 6 in the sequence) should be modified.

5. If the receiver is suffering from any condition, such as dizziness or vertigo, which may be exacerbated by repeated turning movements of the head the massage routine needs to be modified accordingly to take this into account.

6. The client should always be kept warm and well supported under the head and body.

7. Remember to allow the client time to recover after completion of the massage, especially if he/ she feels light headed and then give them a drink of water.

8. The therapist should try to apply the massage with minimum use of the thumbs, posture should be good with body twisting minimised and pressure acceptable for both receiver and therapist.

A Facial Massage Routine

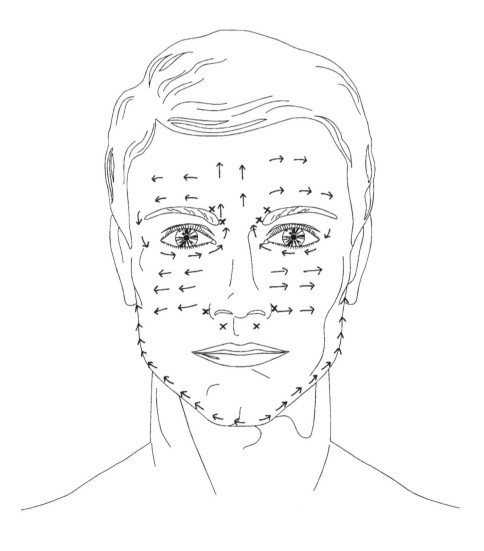

The Face and Neck Sequence

The movements outlined below are a suggested sequence with all major parts of the face and neck being treated, because there are great differences in all therapists' training, skill, experience and techniques it is quite acceptable for different movements to be carried out by different therapists. The important points are to check that the massage is done safely and correctly and that all the necessary areas are treated.

A diagram of the facial part of the sequence is shown in this chapter.

The number of times any movement is repeated is influenced by the condition(s) being experienced by the client. If sinusitis in particular, for example, is being experienced then the sinus drainage areas should be concentrated on by the therapist (nos. 7& 8 in the sequence).

A therapist should try to keep in physical contact with the client all through the massage.

1. Start by holding the sides of the client's head with both hands for a few moments to start contact. Then apply massage cream or oil to the client's forehead, cheeks and throat. If the client prefers, the massage can be done without any medium.

2. Using individual fingers, starting with the first finger, press pressure points of the forehead working up from the eyebrows and just into the hairline, work from centre of forehead across to temples.

3. Stroke across the forehead from the centre of the face to the temples.

4. Circle fingers on temples (clockwise or anti-clockwise).

5. Stroke gently across cheeks several times.

6. Fingertip circle around eye sockets - do not use thumbs to protect them (take care and adjust movement if contact lenses are being worn).

7. Hook in fingers under both cheekbones and firmly slide to ears (first sinus drainage technique).

8. Press points; (i) under centre of nostrils (take care not to press on upper teeth); (ii) 2 points on groove to the side of the nostrils (iii) under eye socket (iv) on forehead in between eyebrows and then (v) squeeze gently eyebrows working outwards (second sinus drainage technique).

9. Run fingers several times up from tip of nose to hairline and then throw over shoulder 'spilt salt throw'

10. Gently squeeze the jawbone from centre of the chin up to the ear and then gently drain down from the ear to the chin on the side of the throat.

11. Gently stroke down sternocleido-mastoid (SC-M) muscle using fingers, thumb or knuckles (use right hand on right side of neck and then left hand on left side of neck) - vary pressure as appropriate. Rest supporting hand on the crown of client's head as a comforter.

12. Gently knead down SC-M with thumb and forefinger; supporting hand remains on crown of head.

13. Massage occipital muscle - the spine is the border, place supporting hand on crown of head.

14. Massage in a circular motion up the neck, decreasing in size until small circles behind ear on the mastoid process, place supporting hand on crown.

15. Place thumb as support behind ear and run forefinger three times up from lobule to helix on outside edge of outer ear.

16. Massage inner part of outer ear with little finger (do not push finger up the outer ear canal) - this stimulates energy points in the ear.

17. Turn head and repeat the previous movements of the other side of the neck.

18. Finally, gently massage the face for a few moments using appropriate movements and finally place hands either over eyes or ears for a short time (this is especially valuable if the therapist is a healer).

After-treatment advice to be offered to the Receiver

It is often very important for a therapist, or medical practitioner, to offer after- treatment advice which will help strengthen the healing process. This is certainly the case with an 'Ear candler' as it is possible that the receiver will not be seen for a period of time, the duration mainly dependant on the remnants of the candles after they have been opened. The advice to be offered is both short term and long term.

Short term advice
- Relax and lie still on the couch for a few minutes
- Get up slowly to avoid an undue draining of blood from the head
- Have a drink of water
- Sit still and do not drive a car or operate heavy machinery for a short length of time. In a noisy environment the noise may be amplified in the short term

- Having used the different session indicators, especially the candles' remnants, advise when the next treatment is due
- Keep the face and neck warm
- If necessary, wear ear plugs when washing, bathing or swimming.

Long term advice
- Have an initial three candles treatments and analyse progress
- If treatments are successful continue, hopefully, on a maintenance basis
- If treatments are unsuccessful go to the GP and ask for tests and procedures to be carried out (possibly in a hospital's ENT/ Audiology Department)
- Keep appointments in the ENT department and accept their help
- Seriously consider vaccinations against disease which may lead to deafness in babies e.g. mumps or measles
- Do not poke or push anything into the ear canal e.g. cotton buds
- Use 5% sodium bicarbonate ear drops to break up ear wax - if there are problems using them, try warmed olive oil or similar
- Wear ear plugs and ear defenders in a noisy or dusty workplace or when carrying out leisure activities like shooting, woodworking and using petrol lawn mowers
- Change diet - increase intake of water, fruit and vegetables; reduce salt, alcohol, caffeine, tobacco and mucous producing dairy foods
- Chew food properly to work the TMJ joint
- Improve lifestyle - eat regularly and get enough sleep
- Reduce stress levels by rearranging work practices and having other therapies such as massage and meditation
- Consider using other treatments and therapies such as osteopathy, chiropractic, acupuncture and reflexology
- Try using a nasal douche if suffering from sinusitis
- Wear wrist pressure bands if suffering from travel sickness
- Join a self help group or support a charity if suffering from a certain condition e.g. Ménière's Society, Tinnitus Association, Defeating Deafness charity etc
- Reduce exposure to loud noise at music concerts - rock, house, classical
- Reduce the use of a personal music player, especially at high volume
- Ensure that silencing on noisy equipment and vehicles is maintained properly
- Keep a diary of events which may trigger conditions such as Ménière's Disease or tinnitus
- Keep hearing aids clean
- Use physical devices which may help socially - special telephones, subtitles on the television, the T-loop hearing aids etc
- Tell others - school, workplace, friends etc if you have hearing or other conditions so that they can help you communicate and have a good social life
- Consider taking Ginkgo Biloba if suffering from tinnitus, as long as it will not contraindicate with other medication.

CHAPTER 2: THE HEAD; ITS PARTS AND HOW THEY WORK

The Skull

The head, or skull, contains the mouth, sense organs and brain. This bony skeleton consists of two parts; the cranium, which surrounds and protects the brain and the facial skeleton.

The cranium consists of eight bones and the face is made up of 14 bones, including the nose, cheeks and jawbones. Immovable joints called sutures fix all the skull bones, except the mandible, to each other. The mandible (the lower jaw bone) articulates with the temporal bones at the freely movable temporomandibular joints (TMJs). The importance of this joint in relation to ear wax expulsion, migraines and snoring is described elsewhere in the book.

Several of the bones are hollow; for example the facial sinus bones whose functions are to reduce the weight of the skull so that it is more easily supported by the spinal column, to protect the brain from damage such as blows or impact, to help with auditory feedback and to condition inhaled air ready for the respiratory process.

Other bones associated with the skull are the hyoid bone, which provides an anchor for the muscles of the back of the tongue, the auditory ossicles which are the three tiny bones in the middle ear and the mastoid bone (which is the lower part of the temporal bone).

The skull also provides attachment points for muscles and helps form the first structural parts of the respiratory and digestive systems.
The skull has a number of cavities;
- the cranial cavity - which houses the brain
- The nasal cavity - smelling and breathing.
- The orbits - which house the eyeballs and eye muscles.
- The mouth.

There are spaces in the temporal bones that house structures of the middle and inner ear.

In the cranium, there are holes for the passage of nerves and blood vessels. Through these pass the cranial nerves (which supply most of the sensory structures and muscles of the head and neck), and blood vessels, such as the carotid arteries and jugular vein, whose function is to carry blood to and from the brain. The largest of these holes is the foramen magnum, which allows the brain stem to enter the spinal canal, where it continues as the spinal cord.

The skull rests on the atlas, which is the first cervical vertebra (bone) which is ring shaped and articulates with the occipital bone at the base of the cranium and allows the head to nod. Turning the head is a function of the joint between the atlas and the axis, which is the second cervical vertebra. The occipital bone, atlas and axis are connected by many small muscles.

Bones of The Skull

Temporal Squamous

Temporal Superior aspect

Temporal Inferior aspect

Coronal Suture

Frontal

Lacrimal

Temporal Fossa

Lamboidal Suture

External Auditory Meatus

Mastoid Process

Maxilla

Zygomatic

Mandible

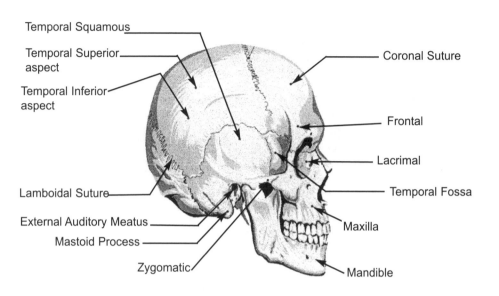

Frontal

Nasal

Parietal

Temporal Squamous

Lacrimal

Zygomatic

Inferior Nasal Concha

Maxilla

Mandible

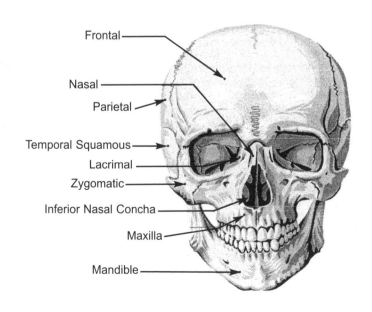

Location of the Facial Sinuses

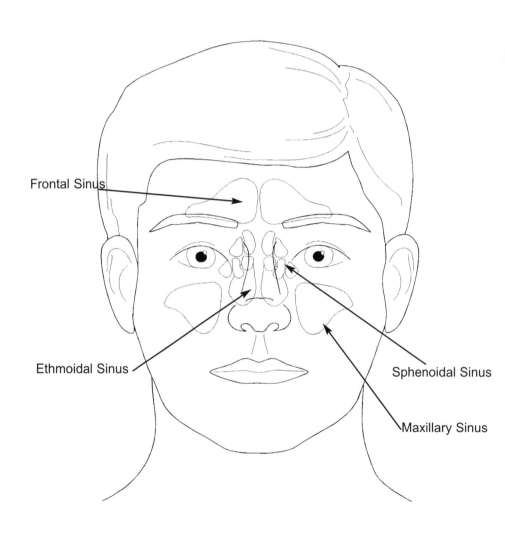

Frontal Sinus

Ethmoidal Sinus

Sphenoidal Sinus

Maxillary Sinus

The skull is covered with skin and hair and is the surrounding structure for the teeth and gums. The blood circulation and lymphatic systems, which are closely linked are also present in the head. Numerous points (nodes) of the lymphatic system are located especially around the ears and jaw bone area (see diagram opposite page 39).

The Facial Sinuses

The Facial Sinuses (Para sinuses), are air filled cavities, lined with mucus membranes, in the bones surrounding the nose, they comprise;
two Frontal sinuses - in the frontal bone of the forehead just above the eyebrows
two Maxillary sinuses - in the cheekbones
two Ethmoidal sinuses - honeycomb - like cavities in bones between the nasal cavity and the eye sockets
two Sphenoidal sinuses - a collection of air spaces in the large winged bone behind the nose that forms the central part of the base of the skull.

Mucus drains from each sinus along a narrow channel, which opens into the nose. Mucus is a thick, slimy fluid secreted by mucous membranes, which as well as being in the respiratory tract is also in the digestive, urinary and genital tracts. The purpose of the fluid is protective by keeping body structures moist and lubricated. It is produced and released on to the surface of the mucous membrane by millions of specialised cells, called goblet cells, which are situated within the membrane itself. The purpose of mucus in the respiratory tract is to moisten inhaled air and to trap smoke and other foreign particles in the airways to prevent them entering the lungs.

The sinuses vary in size; the maxillary being the largest with the volume of a tablespoon. On average the sinus size is 1.25 inches high, 1 inch wide and 1 inch deep. Sinuses are normally bigger in men than women and are less developed in some peoples such as the Maori of New Zealand.

The Brain

The brain has three main parts; the brain stem, the cerebellum and the large forebrain which lies above the brain stem. Much of the forebrain consists of the cerebrum.

The brain is the major organ of the nervous system and while it is the organ of thought, speech and emotion it is more importantly the controlling centre for the body. The brain and spinal cord are the central nervous system (CNS), which controls basic functions such as heart rate, breathing and body temperature. The brain receives and interprets sensations from the nerves that extend from the CNS to every other part of the body. The brain also initiates and coordinates the motor output involved in activities such as movement and speech.

Extending from the brain are 12 pairs of cranial nerves, the most important of these nerves, when talking about the actions of the ear candles treatment are the Olfactory nerve, Trigeminal nerve, Vestibulo-cochlear nerve and the Vagus nerve. All these nerves can be affected by the overall candles treatment, which includes a face and neck massage.

While the complexity of the structure and function of the brain lies outside the scope of this book it is important for the reader to understand how sound is perceived within the brain and this is dealt with in chapter 3. Features associated with parts of the brain which affect hearing, balance, motion, memory and smell are listed below.

The cerebellum is concerned, amongst other things, with balance and posture. It does this by receiving information about the body's position from the ears, eyes and sensory receptors scattered throughout the body in muscles and joints.

Another important part of the brain, the limbic system, which it is believed to be involved in the processing of emotions, some memory functions, and olfactory/smell sensations, is probably affected by the candles through the stimulation of the olfactory nerves and thence to the brain via nerves emanating from the olfactory bulbs.

The other cranial nerves, which are of special interest when considering the candling therapy are the trigeminal nerves (fifth cranial nerve), the facial nerves (seventh cranial nerve) and the vagus nerves (tenth cranial nerve).

The Trigeminal nerve receives sensory impulses of pain, temperature and touch. It also stimulates the muscles of chewing. The ophthalmic branch supplies the lacrimal (tear) glands, the conjunctiva of the eyes, the forehead, eyelids, front of the scalp and the mucous membrane of the nose. The maxillary branch supplies the cheeks, upper gums, upper teeth and lower eyelid. The mandibular branch supplies the teeth and gums of the lower jaw, pinnae of the ears, lower lip and tongue. Motor fibres supply the muscles of chewing.

The Facial nerve has both motor and sensory nerve fibres, the motor fibres supply the muscles of facial expression; sensory fibres convey impulses from the taste buds to the taste perception area in the brain's cerebral cortex.

The Vagus nerve has an extensive network. Motor and sensory nerve fibres supply the smooth muscles and secretory glands of the pharynx, larynx, trachea, heart, stomach, intestines, kidneys, pancreas and many other structures and organs.

The Olfactory nerve is stimulated by odours which are a complex mixture of different compounds, each one at low concentration. Olfactory compounds must contact the nasal mucosa in order to produce a smell and have to be soluble in water and lipids (fat). It is possible to discriminate between many smells at the same time. The olfactory mucosa and pathway rapidly becomes fatigued but recovers quickly.

The Eyes

A detailed description of the structure of the eyes, and conditions generally relating to them are not within the scope of this book. There is one eye condition which has been observed to be affected by the ear candles. This is stimulation of the drainage of the tear ducts, which drain directly into the nasal region.

The eyes are protected by eyelids, which are folds of tissue at the upper and lower edge of the eyes. The eye is the organ of sight. It is constructed so that an image of an object is focused on to the retina, which is at the back of the eye, and nerve cells, which convert this image into electrical impulses. The impulses are carried by the optic nerve for interpretation within the visual cortex of the brain. The optic nerve of each eye meets before they reach the visual cortex. The eyes also have an important input into the processes of balance and motion.

The Nose

The nose is both the upper part of the respiratory tract and also the organ of smell. The structure of the nose is linked to other important areas, which are affected by the action of the ear candles. The nostrils of the nose are connected to the nasopharanx (the upper part of the throat). The nasopharanx is linked to the middle ear via the Eustachian tube.

The bones surrounding the nose contain air filled mucous membrane lined cavities, known as paranasal sinuses, which open into the nasal passage. The nasolacrimal duct, which drains away the tears that bathe and lubricate the front of the eyeball, has an opening in each wall of the nose.

The nose detects smells by the stimulation of hair-like projections from the smell receptors which are situated in the mucous membrane lining the roof of the nose. These olfactory nerve endings, which, when stimulated by inhaled vapours such as those given off when ear candles are burnt, send information to the two olfactory bulbs lying above the bone above the nose and then via the two sensory olfactory nerves to the limbic system and smell centres of the brain.

As well as detecting smells, the nose has several other functions, and these include;

- filtering, warming and moistening inhaled air before it passes into the rest of the respiratory tract
- trapping large dust particles and foreign bodies on the small hairs (cilia) just inside the nostrils and inducing sneezing to remove them
- transporting harmful microorganisms and other foreign bodies towards the nasopharanx so that they can be swallowed and destroyed by the gastric acid in the stomach
- acting as a resonator, helping to give each voice its individual characteristic tone.

Cross Section of the Head and Throat

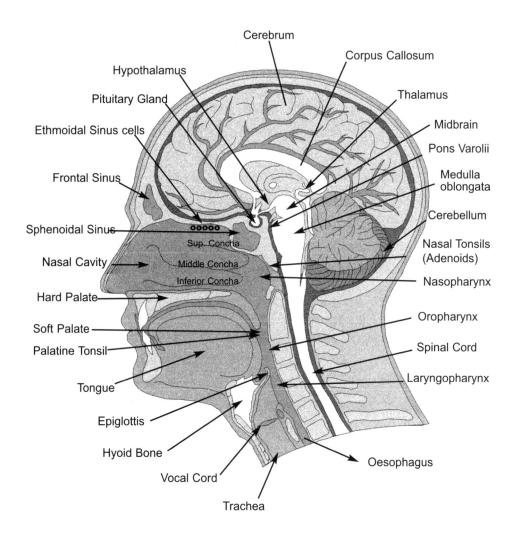

Cerebrum

Corpus Callosum

Hypothalamus

Thalamus

Pituitary Gland

Ethmoidal Sinus cells

Midbrain

Pons Varolii

Frontal Sinus

Medulla oblongata

Sphenoidal Sinus

Cerebellum

Sup. Concha

Nasal Tonsils (Adenoids)

Nasal Cavity

Middle Concha

Inferior Concha

Nasopharynx

Hard Palate

Oropharynx

Soft Palate

Palatine Tonsil

Spinal Cord

Laryngopharynx

Tongue

Epiglottis

Hyoid Bone

Oesophagus

Vocal Cord

Trachea

The Mouth
The mouth or oral cavity is the first part of the digestive system where food is broken down for swallowing. Before food is swallowed it is chewed (masticated); both the tongue and the teeth are active in this process. Saliva contains the digestive enzyme amylase, which helps breakdown carbohydrates. Saliva also contains minerals e.g. sodium, potassium and calcium, various proteins, urea and other ingredients.

The mouth consists of a hard bony palate, the soft fleshy palate, the tongue (containing specialised cells known as taste buds), the teeth, gums and three pairs of salivary glands. The cheeks and lips enclose the structure of the mouth.

The mouth is also used in breathing and converts vibrations, produced by the larynx (voice box), into speech.

The Throat

The throat is the popular term for the pharynx, which is the passage running down the back of the mouth and nose to the upper part of the oesophagus, and the opening into the larynx (voice box). The throat can also be used to refer to the front of the neck. The throat is essential for breathing and eating. It can also change shape and help form vowel sounds. It is a muscular tube with a mucous membrane lining.

The pharynx can be divided into three parts;
- the highest section, the nasopharynx (an air passage) connects the nasal cavity to the area behind the soft palate of the mouth - it is also the bottom end of the Eustachian tube, which connects to the middle ear
- the middle section, the oropharynx (a passage for both air and food) runs from the nasopharanyx to below the tongue.
- the lowest part, the laryngopharynx (a passage for food), lies behind and on each side of the larynx and merges with the oesophagus.

An important structure is the epiglottis, which is a flap of cartilage lying behind the tongue and in front of the entrance to the larynx (voice box). Normally, the epiglottis is upright and allows air to pass through the larynx and into the rest of the respiratory system. During the action of swallowing it folds back to cover the entrance to the larynx, preventing food and drink from being inhaled.

The Voice

The voice is produced by modifying the vibrating column of air from the larynx. The larynx produces the vowel sounds and the pitch and the fundamental frequencies are less than 1,000 Hz (F1: 300-400Hz, F2: 500-1900 Hz, F3 1800-2600 Hz). High frequency sounds are the consonants which are added by the pharynx, tongue, lips and teeth. Quality is added by the nose which allows some air to escape through it.

The sound resonates within the mouth and nose. The nose is most effective when resonating at the laryngeal F1 frequencies. Transmission of sound through the facial skeleton helps monitor voice quality. Many nasal conditions e.g. allergic rhinitis, influenza and nasal polyps affect the quality of the voice by blocking the passage of air on expiration.

Sinuses help with auditory feedback and are unlikely to have any affect on modifying the voice.

The Ears

The ear is the organ of hearing and balance. In chapter 3, we will examine closely the structure of the ear, its functions, and how it relates to other parts of the head. This organ merits special attention as it is the part of the head which is most affected by the use of the ear candles.

Muscles in the Body including the Head and Neck

There are three types of muscle in the body, which are;
●   Skeletal,
●   Smooth,
●   Cardiac.

Skeletal muscle, of which there are more than 600, with many of them being located in the face, are voluntary which means that their action can be consciously controlled. They contain cylindrical cells, which are made up of fibres; each fibre has several nuclei with filaments. When a muscle contracts the filaments slide, which gives a shortening of thickening of the fibres. Most muscles in the face and neck are in this group.

Smooth muscle, these are muscles, which are not under our conscious control. These are found on the walls of blood and lymphatic vessels, in the respiratory, digestive and urinary systems.

Cardiac muscle, powers the pumping action of the heart.

Movement of skeletal muscles is under the voluntary control of the brain. Each muscle fibre has nerve endings, which receive impulse signals from the brain; skeletal muscle activity is affected by changes in chemical composition of the fluid surrounding muscles. A fall in potassium ions causes muscle weakness; a decrease in calcium ions causes muscle spasm.
Smooth, or involuntary muscle has nerve endings in the muscle and they also respond to various hormones, which are produced in the endocrine system. There are also other complex mechanisms such as changes in the chemical composition of fluid surrounding the fibres.

Muscles have to have an adequate supply of blood, which provides oxygen and other nutrients and also removes waste products from energy which is produced within the muscle. Muscles are attached to the rest of the body by ligaments, tendons and the fascia (connective tissue). Ligaments are slightly elastic tissue and attach the same type of structure together, e.g. bone to bone. Tendons are inelastic and extremely strong, they connect muscles with movable structures such as bone, ligaments, cartilage or fibrous membranes. The fascia can either be superficial or deep. The superficial fascia lies beneath the skin and is found over almost the whole surface of the body including the face and neck. It allows the movement of the skin and is the medium of the passage of nerves and blood vessels. Deep inelastic fascia covers muscles and their attachments. It assists muscle action through tension and pressure.

The face and neck massage, which should be carried out as part of the overall ear candles therapy treatment has many aims, which were described fully in chapter 1. One of these aims is to help improve the efficiency of the action of the muscles in this part of the body with the associated increase in activity of the blood and lymphatic systems with the benefits this will bring.

Principal Muscles of the Face and Neck

The Face

There are 97 muscles of the face and it is useful to know the names and function of the principal muscles, which are usually present in pairs one on each side of the face.

Occipitalis - a fibrous sheet over the occipital bone which moves the scalp backwards. This is unpaired

Occipitofrontalis (Occipitalis and **Frontalis)** - lifts eyebrows and wrinkles skin of forehead, which gives the looks of surprise and horror. This is unpaired

Frontalis - fibrous sheet over frontal and parietal bones which moves scalp forwards and raises the eyebrows. This is unpaired

Procerus Nasi - a continuation of the Frontalis down the midline of the nose between the eyebrows. It wrinkles at the bridge of the nose to give a disgusted expression. This is unpaired

Nasalis - at the sides of the nose and compresses and dilates the nasal opening to give an annoyed expression and also sniffing

Levator Labii Superioris - a thin muscular band from the eye to mouth which lifts the upper lip and gives a cheerful expression

Levator Anguli Oris - a thin muscular band of muscle below Levator Labii Superioris which raises the corner of mouth and also produces cheerful expression

Zygomaticus - a thin muscle angled across the face, superficial to Masseter which moves from the angle of mouth upwards, back and out (smiling)

Orbicularis Oris - a sphincter muscle (a muscle with increased number of circular muscle fibres) around the mouth, which purses the lips ready for whistling. This is unpaired

Mentalis - above the tuberosity (a prominent area on a bone, to which tendons are attached) on the chin which lifts the skin on the chin and turns lower lip outwards

Depressor Labii Inferioris - mid-line of the chin to the lower lip which pulls the lower lip down

Depressor Anguli Oris - from Modiolus (of the Cochlea) to Mandible (lower jaw), pulls down corners of mouth

Buccinator - wide thin muscle deep to Masseter. Compresses cheek against teeth to maintain tension (this is known as the 'trumpeter's' muscle!) and also aids mastication (chewing) of food

Risorius - between Masseter and corner of the mouth. Retracts angle of mouth and lifts upper lip which produces a grinning expression

Medial Pterygoid - on the inner surface of the Mandible. Raises Mandible

Lateral Pterygoid - behind the Zygomatic Arch (cheekbone). Pushes Mandible out and closes mouth

Selected Head & Neck Muscles

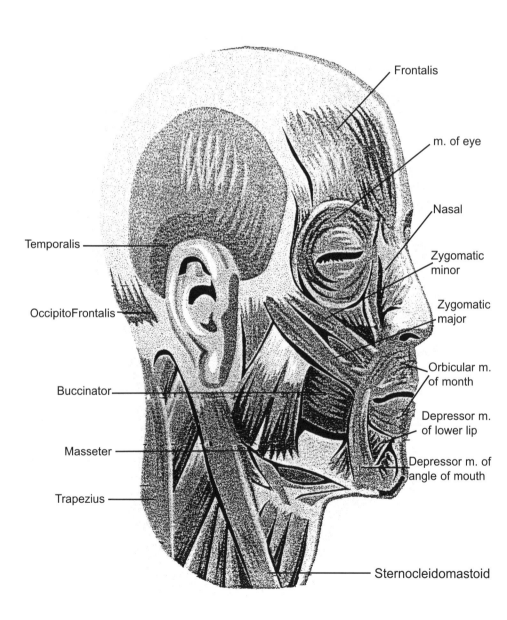

Frontalis

m. of eye

Nasal

Temporalis

Zygomatic minor

OccipitoFrontalis

Zygomatic major

Orbicular m. of month

Buccinator

Depressor m. of lower lip

Masseter

Depressor m. of angle of mouth

Trapezius

Sternocleidomastoid

Masseter - a broad muscle from Zygomatic Arch to Mandible. Raises lower jaw to upper jaw (Maxilla) and exerts great pressure on food
Temporalis - from the temporal bone to the Mandible, it passes behind the Zygomatic Arch, it closes the mouth and helps chewing
Orbicularis Oculi - sphincter muscle around the eye which closes the eyelid and when strongly contracted 'screws up the eyes'
Levator Palpebrae - above upper eyelid. Opens upper eyelid.

The Neck

There are a number of muscles situated in the neck, the three most important to the therapist are;
Sternocleidomastoid muscle - which is rope-like and runs at an angle at the side of the neck, it most importantly flexes the head and allows it to turn from side to side
Trapezius muscle - this covers the shoulder, the back of the neck and the upper back. It is kite shaped and pulls the head backwards, squares the shoulders and controls the movements of the Scapula (shoulder blade) when the shoulder joint is in use
Masseter muscle - as we have seen its action is to raise the lower jaw (Mandible).

It is quite likely that a therapist will work on other muscles situated in the shoulder and upper chest areas when carrying out a neck massage. This is due to the fact that there are linkages between the neck and the shoulder and chest areas.

The Lymphatic system

This is a system of vessels (lymphatics), which drains lymph fluid from all over the body back into the bloodstream and is linked with the blood circulation system. This lymphatic system is part of the immune system and plays a major part in the body's defence against infections.

All bodily tissue is bathed in a watery fluid, which comes from the bloodstream. Much of the fluid returns to the bloodstream through the walls of the capillaries (which link arteries and veins), but the remainder, along with cells and small particles such as bacteria is transported to the heart via the lymphatic system.

Lymph flows through lymph nodes, which filters microorganisms and other foreign bodies contained in the lymph fluid. These nodes generally occur in clusters, mainly around the neck, armpits (Axillary nodes), groin (Inguinal nodes), elbow (Supra-trochlear nodes) and knee (Popliteal nodes). If any part of the body is inflamed or otherwise diseased, the nearest lymph nodes become swollen and tender to limit the spread of the disease. In extreme cases, if infection is particularly virulent the lymphatics may also be inflamed, becoming visible. The nodes contain many lymphocytes (a type of white blood cell), which neutralises or destroys invading bacteria and viruses. The lymphatic system also plays a part in the absorption of fats from the intestine. Other organs which play an important part in the lymphatic system are the spleen, thymus gland, adenoids (especially important in young people) and the tonsils.

Head Lymph Nodes and Vessels

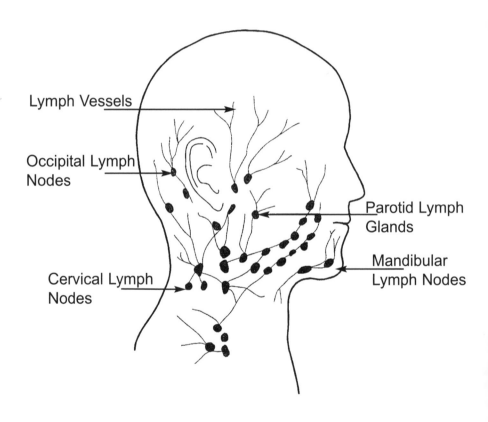

Lymph Vessels

Occipital Lymph Nodes

Parotid Lymph Glands

Cervical Lymph Nodes

Mandibular Lymph Nodes

Just below the neck, the thoracic duct and the right lymphatic duct drain into the two subclavian veins. These veins join to form the inferior vena cava, which passes into the heart - at this point the lymph fluid rejoins the circulation. The position of these major ducts can be taken into account when the therapist carries out the face and neck massage of an ear candles treatment.

The Adenoids

The adenoids are a swelling, consisting of lymph nodes, at the back of the nose above the tonsils. They enlarge during early childhood when infections are common. They normally shrink after five years of age and disappear after puberty.

The Tonsils

This is a pair of oval tissue masses at the back of either side of the throat and consists of lymphoid tissue and like the adenoids form part of the lymphatic system which protects against upper respiratory tract infections. They reach their maximum size at about seven years of age and then shrink away.

Lymphatic nodes are arranged in both deep and superficial groups. Although there are a number of lymph nodes in the face and neck, the most important for the therapist, are the Occipital nodes, Submandibular nodes and the deep and superficial Cervical nodes.

The blood circulation system
The blood circulation system consists of;
- **blood**
- **blood vessels**
- **the heart, which is a pump.**

The blood
Blood has two constituents - plasma, which is a sticky fluid, and cells which float in the plasma. Adults normally have between five to six litres of blood.
Plasma is made up of water and chemical substances dissolved or suspended in the water. The substances are;
- nutrient material absorbed from the intestines
- oxygen which has been absorbed from the lungs
- chemical substances
- waste materials produced by cells, which have to be eliminated from the body.

Blood cells
There are three types of blood cell;
red blood cells (erythrocytes), which carry oxygen within the body and also carbon dioxide between the lungs, and all bodily cells. They contain haemoglobin, which combines with oxygen and is carried from the lungs to the cells.
white blood cells (leukocytes), which mainly protect the body against microbes and other potentially damaging substances, which enter the body. They are also involved with the removal of cells at the end of their normal lifespan and also those damaged by disease and injury. These cells are larger than the red blood cells and are less numerous.

platelets (thrombocytes) are small cell fragments, which play an essential part in the process of blood clotting. A blood clot is a plug of blood cells and fibrous material forming in a cut or torn end of a blood vessel which stops an excessive loss of blood.

Blood vessels

There are three types of blood vessel - arteries, veins and capillaries;

arteries which carry oxygenated blood away from the heart (except the pulmonary artery, which carries deoxygenated blood from the heart to the lungs)

veins which return oxygenated blood to the heart (except the pulmonary veins, which returned oxygenated blood from each lung to the heart)

capillaries which link arteries and veins. These tiny blood vessels have thin walls one cell thick. There are very small openings/pores between these cells, which allow some of the constituents of blood to pass through such as oxygen, nutritional materials, chemical substances and waste products. Larger size substance such as red blood cells and proteins cannot pass through the semipermeable capillary walls. It is through these openings that the aromatherapy ingredients of the ear candles can be absorbed into individual cells of the body.

The Heart

The heart is a fist sized muscular sack which pumps blood into the blood vessels, which transport it to the lungs where oxygen is absorbed from the air and exchange of excreted carbon dioxide (from the blood) into the air is made. The blood is also transported to the individual cells, which make up all parts of the body.

Circulation of blood to the head and neck

The paired arteries, which supply the head and neck, are the common Carotid arteries and the Vertebral arteries. The right common carotid artery is a branch of the brachiocephalic artery. The left common carotid artery rises directly from the arch of the aorta, which in turn leads from the heart. These arteries pass upwards on both side of the neck and have the same distribution on each side. They divide into the external carotid artery and the internal carotid artery from this point. They supply each part of the face and head including the brain.

The External Carotid artery

This artery supplies the superficial tissues of the head and neck and has a number of branches, these are (with their target organs);

superior thyroid artery - thyroid gland and adjacent muscles

lingual artery - the tongue, lining membrane of the mouth, the floor of the mouth, tonsils and the epiglottis

facial artery - muscles of facial expression and structures in the mouth

occipital artery - posterior part of the scalp

temporal artery - frontal/temporal/parietal parts of the scalp

maxillary artery - muscles of chewing and structures in the interior of the skull.

The Internal Carotid artery
This artery supplies the greater part of the brain; it also has branches that supply the eyes, forehead and nose. It is a major contributor to the **Circle of Willis**, which is an intricate system of arteries, which supply most parts of the brain and brain stem.

Return of blood from the head and neck

The venous return of blood from the head and neck is via the deep and superficial veins.superficial veins have the same names as branches of the external Carotid artery and return the deoxygenated blood from the superficial structures of the face and scalp and join to form the external jugular vein. The external jugular vein begins in the neck at the level of the angle of the jaw, it then passes downwards in front of the sternocleidomastoid muscle, and then behind the clavicle (collarbone) before entering the subclavian vein.

The venous blood from the deep areas of the brain is collected into channels, called the dural venous sinuses. There are a number of sinuses, and they join as the internal jugular vein. The internal jugular veins run downwards in the neck behind the sternocleidomastoid muscles behind the clavicle (collarbone). They unite with the subclavian veins, which carry blood from the upper limbs to form the brachiocephalic veins.
The left brachiocephalic vein is longer than the right, and when it joins the right brachiocephalic vein it forms the superior vena cava, which passes down along to the right border of the breastbone (sternum) and ends in the right atrium of the heart.

CHAPTER 3: THE EAR AND HOW IT WORKS

In this chapter as well as looking at the structure of the ear we will examine the physiology/process of its two functions - **hearing and balance**. It will also be useful to explain some of the terms which are commonly used including sound and noise.

HEARING

The parts of the ear

The ear consists of three sections;
●   **the outer ear**
●   **the middle ear**
●   **the inner ear.**

The hearing part of the ear is supplied by the eighth cranial nerve - the cochlear part of the vestibulocochlear nerve, which is stimulated by vibrations initially caused by sound pressure waves from external environmental noise sources.

THE OUTER EAR

The outer ear consists of the **pinna (auricle)** which you can see and is often called the earflap, the curved **external auditory canal (acoustic meatus)** which is the passage along which the sound travels and the **ear drum (tympanic membrane)**.

The pinna

The pinna projects from the side of the head; its body is composed of a thin sheet of fibrocartilage covered with skin and is connected to surrounding parts by ligaments and muscles. It is continuous with the cartilage of the external auditory meatus/ear canal. The cartilage is absent in the lobule and deficient in the upper anterior part where it is replaced by dense fibrous tissue.
It is deeply grooved and ridged and the prominent outer ridge is the helix. The soft, pliable part at the lower end is the lobule, which is composed of fibrous and adipose (fatty) tissue richly, supplied with blood capillaries.
The pinna is covered with fine hairs which have sebaceous glands opening into their root canals. The glands are most numerous in the concha and the scaphoid fossa. Thick hairs may develop from middle age in men on the tragus and intertragic notch. There are three extrinsic muscles which radiate from the pinna; the six small intrinsic muscles serve no purpose except to entertain people when the ear is waggled. The carotid artery serves the pinna and there are many nerves which service it.

The external auditory canal is approximately 2.5 centimetres long and 1 centimetre wide and runs from the concha of the auricle to the tympanic membrane. The lateral (outer) third of the canal is cartilaginous and the rest is in the temporal bone. In adults, the cartilaginous part runs inward, slightly downwards - this is why a medical practitioner has to straighten up the canal by moving the auricle upwards and backwards when using an examination otoscope.

In children, because the ear is not so well developed the auricle is drawn down and backwards to get the best view of the tympanic membrane.

There is a prominence, called the isthmus, which is approximately 5 mm from the tympanic membrane which reduces the canal's diameter.

The skin which lines the canal has lateral growth towards the epidermis and this means that layers of keratin (protein) are shed towards the surface opening of the canal. This process is often found within the epidermal layer of the tympanic membrane and the rate of epidermal migration is about 0.05 mm/day which is the same rate of growth as that of fingernails. The skin which overlays the cartilaginous part contains hairs and glands. The hairs are narrow, short and project towards the canal opening. The external surface of individual hairs has a series of overlapping 'scales' which also direct outwards.

There are two types of glands lining the lateral part of the ear canal;

● **Sebaceous glands**
● **Ceruminous glands.**

Sebaceous glands are similar in structure to comparative glands which are found elsewhere in the body. The central cells which contain fat, break down to form the sebaceous material (sebum) which is replaced by epithelial cells which have proliferated at the edge of the cell mass. Sebum moves along the ducts which nearly always open into hair follicles and as well as waterproofing the skin it acts as a fungicidal and bactericidal agent, which helps prevent the invasion of harmful microbes.

Ceruminous glands lie slightly deeper in the dermis. The contraction of smooth muscle at the base expels the contents of the gland via a duct into the root canal of the hair follicle from which the cells usually originate. The secretion is white and watery but it dries and oxidises, becomes sticky and semisolid and then darkens in colour and can appear to be black in colour when it has been present for some time. The rate of secretion is slightly increased by factors such as emotion, fever, exercise, adrenergic drugs and mechanical manipulation e.g. sticking a finger in the ear canal. As these glands are modified sweat (apocrine) glands they react to stimuli in a similar way as sweat glands.

Ear wax (cerumen)

Although ear wax is dealt with in detail in the next chapter a few words on this phenomenon may be useful. The mixture of the products of the two types of ear canal glands results in ear wax. Types and amount of wax depend on a person's racial origin, occupation, heredity and diet.

Wax contains various amino acids, fatty acids, lysozymes (small molecule proteins with antibacterial properties) and immunoglobulins (antibodies produced to overcome infecting microbes).

Ear hairs

The skin overlying the cartilaginous portion of the ear canal contains hairs (as well as glands). The hairs are narrow, short and point towards the external opening. The hair's surface has a series of overlapping 'scales' which also point outwards. The hairs act as a defensive mechanism to stop objects falling towards the ear drum.

The defensive mechanisms of the outer ear canal

Foreign material, which is potentially damaging such as dirt, insects and microbes should be prevented from reaching the ear drum (tympanic membrane) by;
● the wax - which also combats bacteria and fungi
● the hairs
● the curvature of the ear canal/meatus.

The ear drum (tympanic membrane)

The ear drum is situated at the end of the ear canal and is the junction between the outer ear and the middle ear. Its longest diameter is 9-10 mm and it is a thin, nearly oval disc slightly broader at the top. The malleus/hammer ossicle bone is attached to the membrane on its posterior side. The outer part of the membrane is known as the pars flaccida (loose) and the bulk of the membrane is known as the pars tensor (taut).

The function of the ear drum is associated with all the actions contained within the middle ear.
When sound pressure, which has been externally produced, reaches the ear drum it causes the membrane to vibrate. The membrane has three layers;
☐ an outer covering of hairless skin
☐ a middle layer of fibrous tissue
☐ an inner lining of mucous membrane, continuous with that of the middle ear. Normally, the ear drum is impermeable.

The protective ear wax (cerumen), which has been produced in the ear canal by the two types of gland can be moved away from the ear drum towards the canal opening by two different actions;
☐ by the movements of the temporomandibular joint (the articulation between the mandible and temporal bones) which take place during chewing and talking. These movements 'massage' the cartilaginous meatus, which moves the wax towards the exterior
☐ by the continual epithelial (cell), movement in the skin of the outer ear canal.

THE MIDDLE EAR

The middle ear consists of four parts;
● The Tympanic (tympanum) or middle ear cavity
● The Eustachian tube
● The Ossicles bones -malleus (hammer), incus (anvil), stapes (stirrup)
● The Mastoid air cell system.

The auditory ossicles (bones in the middle ear)

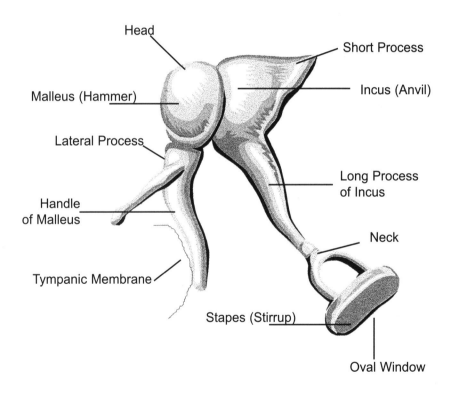

Head

Short Process

Malleus (Hammer)

Incus (Anvil)

Lateral Process

Long Process
of Incus

Handle
of Malleus

Neck

Tympanic Membrane

Stapes (Stirrup)

Oval Window

The Middle Ear Cavity

The middle ear is a space approximately 1.3 centimetres across, which is filled with air. The cavity is irregular - shaped within the petrous/hard portion of the temporal bone and contains the ossicles, two muscles (stapedius and tensor tympani), the chorda tympani nerve and the tympanic plexus of nerves.

One of the main functions of the middle ear is that of impedance/resistance matching. Because the next part of the ear - the inner ear - is filled with fluid while the ear drum is a membrane affected by changes in air/gas pressure there is a large impedance difference which is balanced by the ossicles bones of the middle ear acting as a lever system. The malleus (hammer) bone which is connected to the posterior side of the ear drum experiences large excursions; these are transformed to a much smaller amplitude at the stapes (stirrup) bone which is connected to the much smaller area, in relation to the ear drum, of the oval window generating the much higher pressures suitable for activating the fluid filled inner ear/labyrinth.

The ossicles do not act as an amplifier as no energy is gained in the process; they simply modify the nature of the vibration to maximise the efficiency of the transfer of energy between the outer and inner ear.

The defensive mechanisms in the middle ear

Another important function of the middle ear is to protect the inner ear from particularly large damaging amplitude vibrations (loud noises). This is done as follows;
● the acoustic reflex; this reflex changes the impedance of the middle ear so that it discriminates against large amplitude, low frequency vibrations. This is achieved by contracting the stapedius and tensor tympani muscles which are associated with the ossicles bones. Though mainly a brainstem reflex, this response is affected by the state of an individual's attention
● subluxion of the ossicles; the articular parts of the malleus, incus and stapes bones can move in and out of joint. This subluxion (incomplete dislocation of a joint) reduces the efficiency of the ossicles as a transmission system and so protects the inner ear.

The Eustachian Tube

Air reaches the middle ear cavity by travelling along the Eustachian/auditory (pharyngotympanic) tube (named after Bartolomeno Eustachio, 1520 - 1574, Roman anatomist and surgeon) which extends from the nasopharanyx and thus connects the cavity with the nose and throat. The tube which is approximately 31 - 38 mm long and about 2 mm in diameter in an adult runs forward, downwards and medially from the middle ear and is lined with ciliated epithelium cells. The tube is shorter and straighter in children.

The presence of air at atmospheric pressure on both sides of the tympanic membrane is maintained by the Eustachian tube and this enables the tympanic membrane to vibrate when sound waves strike it. Mostly, the tube is lightly closed but when there is unequal pressure across the membrane it is opened by yawning or swallowing and the ears 'pop' equalising the pressure again.

the lateral wall of the middle ear is formed by the tympanic membrane; the roof and floor are formed by the temporal bone. The posterior wall is formed by the temporal bone with openings leading to the mastoid antrum through which air passes to the mastoid air cells. The medial wall is a thin layer of temporal bone with two openings, the oval window (fenestra vestibuli) and the round window (fenestra cochleae).The oval window is occluded (closed off) by part of the small ossicle bone called the stapes and the round window by a sheet of fibrous tissue.

As well as the proximal bony part of the tube, which is 12 mm in length, the remainder which enters the nasopharynx is comprised of fibrocartilage. The tube is lined with respiratory mucosa containing goblet cells and mucous glands. At the nasopharyngeal end the mucosa is respiratory and the glands and goblet cells decrease towards the middle ear cavity.

The mechanism of tubal opening during swallowing and yawning is not fully understood. The action of the muscles which are attached are incremental especially the tensor tympani, assisted by the tensor veli palatini and possibly the salpingopharyngeus (which is quite slender to have much effect).

The Ossicles bones

A chain of three tiny bones stretch across the middle ear cavity to conduct the sound (vibrations) from the eardrum to the oval window and hence into the inner ear. The bones, the **ossicles;** are called the **malleus** (hammer), the **incus** (anvil) and the **stapes** (stirrup). Their individual size can be likened to a grain of rice.

The malleus (hammer)

This is the largest of the three ossicles and its length is 7.5 - 9.0 mm and has a head, neck and three processes. It is attached to the posterior side of the ear drum and its image can usually be seen during an ear examination using an otoscope. It articulates with the incus bone via an integral synovial joint.

The incus (anvil)

The incus articulates with the malleus and has a body and two processes; its tip articulates with the stapes bone.

The stapes (stirrup)

The stapes has a head, neck, two crura (limbs) and a base/footplate. Its head articulates with the incus and is 2 mm across. The footplate which is attached by an annular (ring-like) ligament to the bony margin of the labyrinthine capsule (the oval window) is 3 mm long and 1.4 mm wide. The stapes is the smallest bone in the body.

Action of sound on the ossicles bones

When sound enters the ear and makes the ear drum vibrate, the vibrations pass from the ear drum along the bones of the ossicles;
☐ the handle of the malleus is in contact with the tympanic membrane (ear drum) and its head forms a movable joint with the incus

46

☐   the body of the incus articulates with the malleus and in turn it articulates with the stapes

☐   the head of the stapes articulates with the incus and it pushes like a little piston against the membrane in the oval window. Behind the oval window is the inner ear.

The three ossicles are held in position by fine ligaments.

The chorda tympani nerve

This branch of the facial nerve enters the tympanic cavity and runs across the medial surface of the tympanic membrane between the mucosal and fibrous layers and passes medial to the upper part of the handle of the malleus bone.

The mucosa (mucous membrane) of the tympanic cavity

The middle ear mucosa is a respiratory mucosa with surface cilia with the ability to be able to secrete mucus. It is more widespread in young people. Mucus fluid comes from goblet cells and mucus glands and can be ejected directly into the middle ear cavity and the Eustachian tube. The mucus membrane lines the bony walls of the cavity and extends to cover the ossicles and their supporting ligaments.

The Mastoid Air Cell System

There are two parts of the system;
●   the aditus to the mastoid antrum
●   the mastoid antrum.

The aditus to the mastoid antrum

This is a large, irregular opening from the posterior epitympanum into the air - filled mastoid antrum; often known as the aditus ad antrum. This structure is very close to the lateral semicircular canal, incus, facial and vestibulocochlear cranial nerves (each only up to 2.36 mm apart).

The mastoid antrum

The mastoid antrum is an air - filled sinus in the petrous part of the temporal bone. It is linked with the middle ear via the aditus and has mastoid air cells arising from its walls. Its volume in an adult is 1 ml; 14 mm from front to back, 9 mm from top to bottom and 7 mm side to side. It is related to different structures including the posterior semicircular canal and the endolymphatic sac. It is situated very close to the brain's temporal lobe.

The mastoid air cell system

In most adults this is a system of interconnecting air-filled cavities which stem from the walls of the mastoid antrum and sometimes the walls of the epi - and mesotympanum. The air cells extend throughout the mastoid process (the part of the bone which can be felt behind the ear).

The internal auditory meatus
This is a short canal almost 1 cm in length which passes into the petrous bone and through which pass the facial, cochlear and vestibular nerves and the auditory artery and vein to and from the cranial cavity.

THE INNER EAR

The component parts of the inner ear have two functions - hearing and balance. It is generally described in two parts;
☐ **the bony labyrinth**
☐ **the membranous labyrinth.**

We have seen that the hearing function of the outer and middle ear is to condition the outside auditory signal arriving at the pinna to make it suitable for the inner ear. In the inner ear the signal (which still consists of rapid pressure change) is processed into a neural code for onward transmission to the brain.

The bony labyrinth

This is a cavity within the temporal bone lined with periosteum (tissue which coats all the bones in the body except the surfaces inside joints). It is larger than, and encloses, the membranous labyrinth.

The labyrinthine fluids

Between the bony and membranous labyrinths is a layer of 'watery' fluid called **perilymph** and within the membranous labyrinth is another 'watery' fluid called **endolymph**. These fluids do not mix.

Endolymph which is thought to be formed in the stria vascularis of the cochlea and also the dark cells of the vestibule, has a high potassium and low sodium concentration and is able to flow between the cochlea and vestibule. A food factor found in tea, coffee and red wine affects the natural movement of endolymph (Harlan and Mann, 1982).

Perilymph has a similar ionic composition to extra cellular fluid and cerebrospinal (CBS) fluid, although there are major differences in the concentration and types of protein present. While the origin of perilymph is unclear it is thought to be produced from cerebrospinal fluid; it could also be a product of ultra filtration through the perilymphatic capillaries (Feldman, 1981).

The bony labyrinth consists of;
● **the cochlea** - the function of hearing
● **the vestibule (saccule and utricle)** - the function of balance and motion
● **three semicircular canals** - the function of rotation and motion.

Together the vestibule and the semicircular canals are known as the vestibular system.

The cochlea

The cochlea is a spiral tube 3.5 centimetres long, which curls 2.75 times. The spiral is divided length wise into three perilymph fluid filled chambers (scala vestibuli, scala tympani and scala media/cochlear duct) which start at the oval window, doubles back and ends at the round window. Sound vibrations pass from the stapes, through the oval window and into the fluid in the outer chamber.

A structure called the basilar membrane performs a mechanical frequency analysis on the incoming signal. This membrane runs almost the length of the cochlea and is narrow at the basal (oval window) end and gradually widens out. Running along this membrane are the rows of hair cells. The short processes of hairs of these cells extend to touch the lower side of the tectorial membrane - a gelatinous shelf which overlies the basilar membrane. Movement of the basilar membrane relative to the tectorial membrane deforms the hairs; it is this deformation which initiates the auditory nerve impulse to the brain.

Subjective Loudness

The amplitude of the response of the basilar membrane to any stimulating sound is not equal for all frequencies. So, sounds of 100 Hz and 1 kHz of equal sound pressure will result in unequal displacements of the basilar membrane. This effect is paralleled in the subjective loudness of the sounds - 100 Hz sound will appear quieter than the sound at 1 kHz.

The vestibule

The vestibule (saccule and utricle) is approximately the size of a pea (5 mm high, 5 mm long and 3 mm deep) and is the expanded part of the labyrinth nearest the middle ear, it contains the round and oval windows in its lateral wall. The vestibule plays an integral part of the function of balance and motion.

The three semicircular canals

The semicircular canals are three tubes (superior, posterior and lateral) arranged so that one is in each of the three planes of space. They are contiguous with, above and behind, the vestibule. Each is two-thirds of a circle and while being unequal in length their lumen has a diameter of approximately 0.8 mm.
At one end of each canal is a dilation called an ampulla which contains the vestibular sensory epithelium and it opens into the vestibule.
The canals' function is to be an important part of the balance and movement processes which are described later in this chapter.

The membranous labyrinth

It is the same shape as the bony labyrinth, is separated from it by perilymph and contains endolymph fluid which is produced by the secretory cells of the stria vascularis of the cochlea and the dark cells of the vestibular labyrinth. It is suspended by fine connective tissue strands from the bony labyrinth and has the same parts as the bony labyrinth;

☐ **one cochlea**
☐ **one vestibule (saccule and utricle)**
☐ **three semicircular canals.**

49

The central chamber of **the cochlea** (within the membranous labyrinth) contains up to 35,000 specialised cells, which resemble microscopic hairs of differing lengths, in the spiral **organ of Corti**, which is contained in the basal membrane. These cells translate vibrations, which are activated by the endolymph fluid, into nerve impulses. These impulses are then transmitted via the cochlear nerve through the brain stem and into the acoustic imaging centres in the cerebral cortex of the opposite temporal lobe. The medial areas are responsible for high frequency recognition and the more lateral areas of the cortex are responsible for low frequency recognition.

The saccule lies in a recess near the opening of the scala vestibuli part of the cochlea (to which it is connected) and is almost globular shaped. It is also connected to the endolymphatic duct and contains an anterior vertical wall of **macula** - a thickened area of sensory epithelium.

The utricle which is irregularly oblong in shape is larger than the saccule and lies above and behind it. The three semicircular canals open into it via five openings (the posterior and superior canals sharing one opening at the crus commune). On its floor lies the sensory epithelium of the comma-shaped macula.

The three semicircular canals are small and ring- like; each forming two - thirds of a circle with a diameter of approximately 6.5 mm and a luminal cross section diameter of 0.4 mm. One end of each canal is dilated/swollen to form the ampulla, which contains a saddle shaped ridge - the **crista ampullaris**, on which the sensory epithelium lays.

Sensory epithelium is localised to the **maculae** (small areas of sensory epithelium) of the utricle and saccule and the cristae ampullaris of the semicircular canals. The sensory hair cells are surrounded by supporting cells. Close to the sensory epithelium are the dark cell regions which are thought to secrete the vestibular endolymph and contribute to its electrical potential.

Vestibular receptor cells

There are approximately 23,000 hair cells in the three cristae of the semicircular canals and between 45,000 and 60,000 in the two maculae of the vestibule. The vestibular hair cells can be generalised into 2 types; type I which are flask- shaped and type II which are cylindrical They both have a basal nucleus but different type of nerve synapse.

The process (physiology) of hearing

Sound

Physically, sound is any undulatory motion in an elastic medium (gaseous, liquid or solid) which is capable of producing the sensation of hearing. The normal medium is air.

Noise

Noise, on the other hand, may be subjectively defined as a sound which is unpleasant, distracting, uncalled for or otherwise undesirable. The human hearing mechanism has a wide range and is quite tolerant; if the tolerance is exceeded there may be the following effects;

● the hearing mechanism may be damaged, temporarily or permanently, including partial deafness or a noise induced temporary threshold shift (TTS)
● communications may deteriorate
● noise may be stressful and this may induce fatigue and other symptoms
● tinnitus (ringing in the ear) which can be caused by a continued firing of the auditory nerve.

Aspects of Sound

Every sound produces sound waves (vibrations) which are compressed and rarefied in the air. A simple sound in which the pressure fluctuations follow a sinusoid is known as a pure tone.

The velocity with which the waves of compression and rarefaction move is called the velocity of sound. The frequency of the sound is the number of times with which each complete cycle repeats itself in a given time. The wavelength is the distance between two corresponding points in successive cycles so -

$$\text{Wavelength} = \frac{\text{Velocity}}{\text{Frequency}}$$

Sound Pressure

In a pure tone, the sound pressure fluctuates so that for half the time it is above, and for half the time below, atmospheric pressure. The sound pressure can be specified in terms of the amplitude - the peak value of each half cycle. Normally it is specified as the average pressure throughout the cycle even though it is fluctuating about prevailing atmospheric pressure. The ear has a very wide dynamic range.

Sound Pressure Level

Because the ear has a large dynamic range and because it responds to changes in a relative, rather than an absolute way, it is convenient to use a scale based on the logarithm of a ratio such as the decibel (dB). Its calculation for any sound is based on the starting point of absolute sound pressure which approximates to the threshold of human hearing at 1 kilohertz (1 kHz).

An increase in sound pressure level of 20 dB equates to a ten-fold increase in sound pressure. Examples of sound pressure levels (dB) on an A weighting include;

● 0 dB (A) - threshold of hearing at 1 kHz
● 40 dB (A) - noise in a library
● 60 dB (A) - ordinary spoken conversation
● 80 dB (A) - street corner traffic noise and normal speech at 3 feet away
● 120 dB (A) - large jet landing
● 140 dB (A) - turbojet at 50 feet away and the threshold of pain.

Measurement of sound level

A sound level meter consists of a microphone, an amplifier and a voltmeter. The voltmeter is graduated in decibels. The instrument is set up so that responses to various sound pressure levels are the same at all frequencies, when it can be used to measure sound pressure level.

In order to make measurements of sound levels which approximate to their subjective loudness a weighting network is used to modify the linear response of the standard setting of the meter The weighting scales are 'A', 'B' and 'C'.

Complex Sounds

A finite signal no matter how complex may be considered to comprise a number of simple sine waves (Fourier series). The sine wave components of a signal constitute the frequency spectrum. The frequency spectrum of a sine wave is only one line; that of more complicated but periodic waves consists of harmonically related discreet lines; that of statistically distributed signals e.g. random noise, shows a continuous spectrum.

If two pure tones are played together they are heard subjectively as a chord rather than a single note - the ear is performing a Fourier analysis on the signal.

The Hearing Journey

Sound pressure waves are vibrations which travel through the air at about 332 metres (1088 ft.) per second, the velocity of sound through water is about 1,425 metres (4,700 ft.) per second. The journey of sound is thus;

☐ the auricle's shape directs the sound waves along the ear canal, which causes the ear drum to vibrate in response to changes in air pressure in the ear canal. The ear drum has a certain resistance to movement (impedance) and the canal performs significant matching of this impedance to the air. The matching is quite frequency dependent, being poor at frequencies below 400 Hz, which is not very important in the comprehension of speech

☐ vibrations are transmitted across the middle ear through the movement of the three ossicles (the first of which, the hammer, is attached to the ear drum)

☐ the foot plate of the stapes bone rocks to and fro in the oval window, setting up fluid waves in the perilymph in the inner ear/labyrinth

☐ the waves indent the membranous labyrinth causing a wave motion in the endolymph (the inner fluid), which stimulates the neuroepithelial cells of the spiral organ of Corti. These nerve impulses pass to the brain in the cochlear portion of the vestibulocochlear nerve (the eighth cranial nerve)

☐ The nerve impulses are sent through the brain stem and into the acoustic imaging centres in the cerebral cortex of the opposite temporal lobe. Medial areas being responsible for recognition of high frequency and the more lateral cortex areas are responsible for low frequency recognition.

☐ the fluid wave is finally expended against the middle ear by vibration of the membrane of the round window.

Sound Action and Reaction within the Cochlea

When movement of the stapes bone, which is attached to the outside of the labyrinth at the oval window, causes pressure changes in the endolymph of the scala vestibuli (these are at the same frequency as the sound arriving in the ear and proportionate to amplitude) a travelling wave is produced in the basilar membrane. This travelling wave starts initially as a bulge at the membrane's basal end and over the next four milliseconds it travels along the membrane, waxing and waning. The point at which the maximum amplitude of vibration occurs on the basilar membrane depends on the stimulating sound's frequency. Low tones produce maximum excitation at the basal end and high tones at the apex.

The information relayed to the brain via the auditory nerve is not only dependant on the location of maximum vibration on the basilar membrane; the frequency of impulses in any nerve fibre or collection of fibres corresponds to the frequency of the stimulating sound. This relationship holds for frequencies up to 3-4 kHz, the highest frequencies used in speech. So there are two ways in which the frequency of the sound is indicated to the brain;
● the rate of firing of the auditory nerve
● the exact location of maximum displacement of the basilar membrane.

The cochlear part of the vestibulocochlear nerve transmits the impulses to the hearing area of the cerebrum where sound is perceived and to various nuclei in the pons varolii in the mid brain.

Sound waves have property of pitch and volume; when sound waves enter the cochlea fluid they move the hair cells and these send electrical messages to the auditory nerve. Different sound frequencies are picked up by hair cells of differing length, depending on their location in the cochlea spiral tube. Short fibres are activated by high frequency sound, medium fibres are activated by medium frequency and long fibres are activated by low frequency. The shorter hair cells are proximal (nearest) to the oval window.
The nerve then passes afferent impulses up to the brain (each cochlear nerve has about 30,000 myelinated nerve fibres), which recognises them as different sounds, for example people crying or doors squeaking.

BALANCE AND MOTION

The **three semicircular canals** and the **vestibule** are the structures of the inner ear which are collectively known as the **vestibular system** and are concerned with balance and motion.

The vestibular system;
● detects body motion (linear and angular acceleration) as monitored by head motion
● detects the position of the head in space relative to the gravitational vector (tilt).

This information is integrated with other inputs for;
● the maintenance of the head on the object of visual fixation
● the maintenance of balance

- the activity of the autonomic nervous system
- the level of arousal and mood

The three semicircular canals are membranous ducts containing the same endolymph and perilymph fluid found in the cochlea. They too have an outer bony wall and membrane which separates the two fluids. Each has a swelling (the ampulla) where the sensory cells are congregated in a ridge (the crista). These cells have many hair-like projections arising from them and are covered by a gelatinous/jelly structure **(the cupula)**. They do not have hair cells, but structures, called **ampullas**. The canals contain the sensory receptors which respond specifically to angular accelerations.

The cupula fills a cross-section of the ampulla and can be likened to a watertight swing door which is deflected by movement of the endolymph within the membranous duct. The activity of the sensory cells is determined by the bending of the hair-like processes which are in turn dependent on the position and movement of the 'swing door' cupula.

The sensory cells in the ampulla of each semicircular canal are maximally stimulated by angular acceleration in the specific plane of the canal. The three canals in each ear are approximately at right angles to each other. An angular acceleration in any plane will stimulate at least two canals in each ear.

The vestibule consists of two endolymph sacs - the **saccule** and the **utricle** which lie below the semicircular ducts and contain sensory cells - the maculae. It also houses the otolithic sense organs which are the receptors of linear accelerations of the head. Sensory hairs signal the position of the head with respect of the gravitational vertical.

There are two otolithic containing organs on each side of the head; those in the utricle lie approximately horizontal when the head is the normal upright position and those in the saccule lie in the vertical plane. This arrangement allows the brain to sense a linear acceleration in any direction. The microscopic chalk otoliths (ear stones) should be embedded in a jelly like substance and weigh it down and help the ear to be sensitive to gravity. If fragments of the crystals, which are being constantly formed/reabsorbed/reformed, break off and fall into one of the three semicircular canals (which are responsible for sensing rotation) movement in that canal will cause the fragment to move, stimulate the canal and give rise to a feel of rotation and a bout of BPPV (Benign Paroxysmal Positional Vertigo).

In the walls of the utricle and the saccule are fine hair cells which have the microscopic nerve endings of the vestibular part of the vestibulocochlear nerve.

The vestibular system control of the muscles is complex and this includes a powerful control over the eye muscles. The vestibular reflex stabilises the position of the eye, relative to an object fixed in space, when the head moves. So, when the head is suddenly moved, the eye is reflex moved in the opposite direction in order to stabilise the image of the outside environment on the retina.

The process (physiology) of balance

Any change in the head's position causes movement in the endolymph and perilymph fluids, which in turn stimulates the nerve endings in the vestibule. The resultant nerve impulses are transmitted to the vestibular nerve which joins the cochlear nerve to form the vestibulocochlear cranial nerve. The vestibular branch first passes to the vestibular nucleus and then to the cerebellum part of the brain.

The vestibular nerve has a smaller number of afferent nerve fibres transmitting information to the brain (19,000-20,000) than the cochlear nerve. It does contain a greater number of efferent nerve fibres.

The cerebellum also receives nerve impulses from the eyes and sensory (moving towards the brain) receptors (proprioceptors) in the skin, muscles and joints. Impulses from the three sources are co-ordinated and efferent (moving away from the brain) nerve impulses pass to the cerebrum where position in space is perceived and also to skeletal muscles, so maintaining body balance and posture.

CHAPTER 4: EAR WAX

Introduction

The subject of ear wax (cerumen) which is a natural protective bodily substance, and its production and cleansing, has been discussed since the ancient times of the Egyptians and Assyrians. Because many people find this substance fascinating I thought it would be useful to devote a chapter of this book to it. Greater knowledge of its function should help dismiss some of the myths which surround it.

The meaning of the word cerumen, which is often used as a synonym for ear wax is derived either from the Latin word cera (meaning wax) or the Greek words keros (meaning wax) or keroumenos (meaning formed of wax).

Ear wax, while seeming to have a simple appearance, has in fact a complex structure. Treatments for excessive and/or impacted wax have usually been one of the following;

☐ mechanical removal such as ear irrigation (previously known as ear syringing)
☐ introduction of a natural product such as a warmed olive oil
☐ use of a commercial organic solvent such as Cerumenex
☐ a combination of the above treatment methods.

The ear candles treatment is becoming increasingly popular, especially with those unfortunate people who have suffered when undertaking one of the more traditional treatment methods. It should be emphasised that any wax found in a used candle's filter is beeswax and not ear wax.

The function and composition of ear wax

Ear wax (cerumen) is a mixture of secretions from two different types of gland - ceruminous (which produces cerumen) and sebaceous (which produces sebum (an oily secretion)). These substances are deep in the lining of the skin in the approximately outer third portion of the auditory meatus/external auditory canal together with epithelium scales (squames), keratinocytes, dust and other foreign matter such as insects. Cerumen also contains other substances; the most important of which are fatty acids, which inhibit the growth of fungi and bacteria.

The secretion of cerumen is similar to the process of the axillary sweat glands - hence there can be some odour. A possible irritation of the overlying skin causes surrounding myoepithelial cells to contract so expelling liquid contents into the outer part of the ear canal. These cells are known as goblet cells. Evaporation then occurs and the now sticky substance traps foreign objects such as dust, fungus and bacteria before they are expelled by the processes of epithelial migration enhanced by movements of the jaw joint (temperomandibular joint (TMJ)).

The quantity of ear wax produced varies between individuals. Many people working or living in a dusty or noisy environment or who may be under stress produce a large amount of protective ear wax. The question of heredity may be relevant and it is likely that those who have their ear wax removed by medical irrigation will produce more wax to replace that which has been removed.

The composition of cerumen varies according to racial grouping. Most Caucasians and Negroes have a 'wet' phenotype with moist sticky, honey (yellowish brown) coloured cerumen. The Japanese, other Mongoloid races and Native American Indians on the other hand mainly have grey or yellow, granular and brittle cerumen - the 'dry' phenotype.

The type of wax is probably monofactorially inherited with the wet phenotype dominant over the recessive dry type. The factor of diet should also be taken into consideration as the staple diet of the Japanese and other Eastern people is rice; white and black people generally have a staple of potatoes and wheat. The question of people originating from the Indian sub-continent is interesting as those from the north predominately consume wheat and those in the south rice.

Wax may reflect disease or condition. With cystic fibrosis, for example, the cerumen is little and dry. Psoriasis can sometimes cause an increase in waxy material because the proliferation of the cells of the basal layers have a rapid upward progress through the epidermis especially in periods of a condition's activity.

Symptoms of wax impaction

There are many symptoms of ear wax impaction, these include;

☐ pain
☐ deafness,
☐ tinnitus
☐ inflammation of the meatal skin of the external ear canal (Otitis externa)
☐ reflex cough
☐ earache
☐ vertigo (a severe form of dizziness).

If the wax is obscuring the ear drum (tympanic membrane) diagnosis of problems can be confused. Although it can be said that any improvement of hearing is subjective once earwax has been removed there can be an improvement in hearing. In Scotland in 1990 a survey (Sharp J F et al) showed that a 5db (decibel) improvement had been achieved over frequencies analysed after ear syringing had taken place. Wax can often reduce the efficiency of hearing aids and for this reason wax guards have been introduced to reduce the damage being caused to receivers by the presence of excessive wax.

If the ear drum is allowed to be obscured by wax and other debris as well as leading to a possible hearing loss there is a danger of ear drum perforation if there is a sufficient increase of pressure on the membrane. This condition is called Keratosis obturans and is often associated with bronchiectasis (a lung disorder, which is sometimes seen as a complication of cystic fibrosis) and sinusitis especially in younger people.

A reflex secretion of wax in the meatus can be caused by the irritation of the efferent vagal nerve endings in the bronchi (in the lungs).

Other than the ear's own natural methods of moving cerumen along the ear canal towards the entrance of the ear, namely the action of the TMJ and epithelial migration there are two main medical processes for the removal of ear wax, these are;

☐ **by mechanical means such as ear irrigation** (usually following the use of appropriate ear drops to soften ear wax) by trained medical staff such as the Practice Nurse at a GP surgery

☐ **by the administration of a ceruminolytic liquid solution to disintegrate the wax** which will later spontaneously leave the ear canal.

History of the treatment of excessive ear wax

Historically, there have been a number of different recommended materials to remove earwax and these have included;
the ancient Assyrians - application of oil of Cedar tree or oil of Cypress tree together with the consumption of wheaten bread and mustard with pomegranate water. If there was hearing loss, some of the following could be inserted in the ear - pig's fat, cat's blood, human semen or a male bat's head (presumably grated)
1705 - Grau recommended olive oil as the preferred ceruminolytic
1860 - Toynbee preferred sodium bicarbonate
1973 - Paparella recommended Cerumenex or hydrogen peroxide
1976 - Hinchcliffe recommended olive oil
1983 - Maran recommended sodium bicarbonate and glycerine.
While some research recommended certain products other research has concluded that certain agents are 'useless' e.g. in 1968 Horowitz concluded that olive oil was useless, and Waxsol was the only product of any value.

Research papers produced at the University of Toronto in 1989 and 1990 (by Robinson A C et al) compared the efficiency of the various ceruminolytics which were then available; the composition of ear wax 'plugs' and the process by which the plugs are broken down or disintegrated.
Some proprietary remedies, which are available without prescription, merely soften and lubricate the wax prior to irrigation; other preparations completely dissolve and liquefy wax and no irrigation will be necessary.
The researchers found that **the best results** were gained from (in ranking);
☐ sodium bicarbonate (5% solution)
☐ sodium bicarbonate (10% solution)
☐ glycerine.
The first two solutions are aqueous (water) based.

Often the wax will swell up after application of the ceruminolytic usually in drops and the patient should be warned that there might be a temporary diminution (reduction) of their hearing and the reason for it occurring.
The researchers questioned the availability and continued use of most organic based commercial ceruminolytics.
The question of administering sodium bicarbonate ear drops has to be considered carefully when treating someone suffering from Ménière's Disease as the introduction of sodium into his/her diet is discouraged. Some young children and senior citizens especially and others may have an intolerance to the use of sodium bicarbonate and if this is the case then an alternative such as warmed olive oil should be considered.

How do efficient aqueous based ceruminolytics work?

The Toronto researchers found that the desquamated (shed) sheets of corneocytes from the skin's stratum corneum (surface, horny layer) are the major constituents of wax plugs and provide the framework for the wax bolus. Ceruminolytics work by hydrating (adding water to) the keratin (fibrous protein) cells, which form 60% of the sheets, with subsequent induced keratolysis (breaking up) and associated wax disintegration.

The researchers also found that;

● impacted cerumen/wax plugs consist of large sheets of keratin which have not separated by normal mechanisms

● hard wax plugs contain more keratin than soft cerumen plugs - these are recognisable by the browner colour of the wax. In soft plugs the sheets of keratin have a large number of corneocytes that have undergone expansion.

Research at the University of Pittsburgh, USA

In 1991, researchers in Pittsburgh reported that they had found that docusate sodium, which is commonly used as a stool softener, to be a highly efficient ceruminolytic agent. It is contained in Waxsol, a proprietary brand and is helpful in three ways;

☐ it softens impactions which proved resistant to instrument or lavage (water) removal

☐ it softens hardened debris in a mastoidectomy cavity

☐ it prevents impactions with bimonthly use.

Waxsol is usually used as a precursor to 'ear irrigation'.

Current methods of removing ear wax

There are four main conventional methods of removing ear wax which is impacted in the external auditory canal especially when it is attached to the eardrum. These are;

☐ irrigation (formerly 'syringing') of the wax bolus, and other methods of lavage

☐ removal using a variety of wax curettes, wire loops or probes

☐ suction debridement, especially by a hospital specialist

☐ application of a ceruminolytic solution.

'Ear irrigation'

Ear irrigation has superseded ear syringing in most cases but it may still take place. Syringing was a common minor procedure, carried out in general practice or in the office of a primary care physician; it was often delegated to the Practice Nurse. It was conducted with great care because of potential risks if recommended procedures were not adhered to such as ear drum perforation or outer ear canal infections and had the following contraindications;

☐ presence of infection in the ear canal

☐ the ear drum had a perforation or it was suspected that the ear drum was vulnerable

☐ a grommet, or other drainage device, is present in the ear drum

☐ any history of problems arising after previous 'syringing'.

In 1990, in the Scottish Lothian district served by 312 General Practitioners with a population of 650,000 approximately 44,000 ears were syringed, and from this number 44 complications had to be referred further to hospital specialists for treatment. Extrapolated nationally this would have given a figure of almost 4,000 referrals.

The new procedure of ear irrigation is safer and can cause less discomfort to the patient as it is gentler in its action. It is more fully described in chapter 7.

Other forms of water treatment

In the United States, dental oral jet irrigators have been adapted for the removal of ear wax. Because of the power of these jets, which is greater than the traditional syringing machines, extreme care has to be taken and strict guidelines have to be followed such as using the lowest power setting and the tip should have multiple orifices.

Mechanical aids
General practitioners and their nurses can use mechanical aids to help remove debris - including the Jobson Horne probe, Cawthorne wax hook or Tilley's dressing forceps. Obviously, great care has to be taken to avoid perforation or the tearing of skin.

Suction debridement or microsuction

This is a highly skilled procedure, which is carried out by a specialist, usually in a hospital's Ear Nose and Throat department. The author was able to observe microsuction taking place in a hospital ENT department and the procedure which 'hoovered out' deeply impacted black ear wax was much more successful than ear irrigation on the same patient carried out a short time before in a GP practice.

Ceruminolytics

We have already looked at this type of material in depth. However, it should be remembered that some of their ingredients could be skin irritants and they should not be used for more than a few days before wax removal, especially with the organic solvents group. If a medical practitioner recommends their use, the length of time before the patient has to return for ear irrigation will be advised. In extreme cases reaction to ceruminolytics may cause Otitis externa, which can lead to severe pain. Two major irritants were found in Cerumol and a skin sensitiser in Auralgan. If these ingredients lead to inflammation in the ear canal skin this could be a cause of contact dermatitis (Robinson A C, Hawke M 1989).

Do-it-yourself home mechanical methods

There are numerous items that people have inserted in their ears to try to remove debris including wax. The most common are fingers, cotton buds, wood, pencils, knitting needles and plastic pen caps. It is not advisable to introduce these items because;

☐ they can introduce infection
☐ they can break and become lodged - often broken items are found years later
☐ they can damage the skin or ear drum
☐ they can impact debris or wax further down into the ear canal towards the ear drum.

There is an old proverb which says that 'nothing smaller than the elbow should be placed in the ear'!

CHAPTER 5: EAR PROBLEMS
Introduction

In this chapter we will look at a number of the conditions which affect the ears; in subsequent chapters we will look at the wide range of preventative methods which can be adopted and the different types of treatments which can be undertaken. The enormity of the problem can be gauged from statistics such as 8.7 million people in the UK are deaf or hard of hearing (Royal National Institute for Deaf and Hard of Hearing People (RNID)) or 80% of all pre-school children will suffer from glue ear (Defeating Deafness).

As we have seen the ear has two functions; hearing and balance. The ears carry out the function of hearing and the brain acts upon the messages sent up the acoustic nerve. With balance, the ear is linked to the brain via the vestibular nerve. The brain also receives information from receptors in other parts of the body - the eyes, skin, muscles and joints.

Because of the complexity of the ear, and the great number of conditions which may affect it, in this chapter we will only be considering the more common problems of the ear.

HEARING PROBLEMS

There are two main categories of hearing impairment, or deafness;
Conductive
Sensorineural (perceptive)
There can be a third category which is mixed hearing loss which includes otitis media and otosclerosis.

Conductive deafness/hearing impairment

Conductive deafness is normally caused by problems;
☐ in the outer ear - which is the part of the ear (the external auditory meatus) which runs from the external Pinna/Auricle to the ear drum
☐ in the middle ear - which is the (post) tympanic cavity behind the ear drum, the Eustachian tube and the three ossicle bones.

The outer ear

The main problem which causes hearing impairment in the outer ear is a blockage occurring in the external curved ear canal. A blockage can be caused by excessive ear wax, which in extreme cases can be a solid plug formed right up to the entrance to the canal. Normally however, wax if it is blocking the eardrum will only reduce the amount of sound by up to five dbA (decibels). If wax is impacted on the ear drum the drum will not vibrate properly and sound will not be transferred through to the ossicle bones behind the ear drum.

Some wax is needed as a protective mechanism. It is possible that by changing elements of diet, such as reducing the intake of fatty foods (which influence the activity of the cells lining the canal) and dairy products which are known to stimulate mucus production this may reduce the amount produced; conversely an increase in exercise may increase its production. In a 'healthy ear canal' wax should only be present in the outer third of the ear canal where the producing glands are situated.

In a dusty or dirty environment the protective action of wax is more essential so more is likely to be produced. To reduce the need for surplus wax, which has been produced because of environmental reasons, the wearing of clean efficient ear protectors, such as earplugs or earmuffs especially in the workplace is essential. Even at home, ear defenders should be used when undertaking noisy activities; such are shooting, drilling, sawing or cutting grass with a petrol mower for a length of time.

It seems logical that if all the wax is removed from the ear canal then the body will be stimulated to produce more replacement wax. If imbalances in diet, environment or activities are predisposed to produce excess wax the cycle of problems needing treatment will continue.

Other blockages in the ear canal can be foreign bodies such as insects, seeds, fragments of building materials and items which may have been placed there on purpose, such as cotton buds, stones and toys. The warm, moist and dark canal is an attraction for insects, especially in warm climates. Seeds have been known to swell in the canal and if this happens, medical attention should be sought.

Outer ear canal infections

Infection in the outer ear canal (otitis externa) can be diffused or localised, unilateral or bilateral with symptoms including itching, pain, discharge and mucus. It can take the form of an abscess. Earache can be accompanied by irritation in the outer ear canal, discharge and slight hearing loss. It can be caused by;
- trauma - scratching
- infection - dirty water, dust or a foreign body
- skin disease - eczema, psoriasis, herpes zoster or impetigo
- allergy - antibiotics or metal (e.g. ear rings, studs).

Skin Conditions

As well as skin cancers, the pinna and outer ear canal are affected by several skin conditions, especially psoriasis, dermatitis and eczema;

☐ **Psoriasis** causes patches of inflamed red skin often covered by silvery scales. New skin cells are produced much faster than normal, with live cells forming patches covered with dead skin. Attacks are of varying severity with periods of remission in between; they may be triggered by a number of factors including emotional stress, skin damage and illness

☐ **Dermatitis** is an allergic reaction condition. There are red, itchy patches, which may cause blisters or crusts. In the ear the reaction is usually to cosmetics, hats or cheap jewellery (such as earrings). Often it is only skin tests which will identify the exact ingredient to which the ear is allergic

☐ **Eczema** is an inflammation which usually causes itching and sometimes scales and blisters. It can sometimes be caused by an allergy but often occurs for no reason. There can be periods of remission between attacks. Often, sufferers may have other allergies, such as asthma or rhinitis

☐ **epidemic cysts and lesions** are located on the pinna, normally on the lobe and are caused by a reaction to jewellery, especially cheap nickel earrings and studs.

The Middle Ear

Conductive hearing loss in the middle ear is either associated with infection in the Eustachian tube and (post) tympanic cavity or problems with the ear drum or three ossicle bones when they do not work properly.

Middle ear infections

There are several types of middle ear infections. The most common are Otitis media and Otitis media with effusion ('Glue ear').

Otitis media

Otitis media is inflammation of the middle ear/ (post)tympanic cavity. Inflammation occurs as a result of a viral or bacterial upper respiratory tract infection, extending up the Eustachian tube. The tube may become blocked by the inflammation or sometimes by enlarged adenoids. Adenoids are lymph nodes, which contain white cell lymphocytes, which help fight infection as part of the immune system. Normally in children, adenoids shrink after five years of age but they can enlarge and they can block the passage from the nose to the throat.

Glue ear

Symptoms of Glue ear

Because it is so common, especially in children, glue ear merits special mention. If glue ear is severe there can be a hearing loss of up to 50db (A) which has serious implications socially and educationally, especially for children who are the most common sufferers of this condition because their Eustachian tube is shorter and straighter than an adult's so they are more susceptible to infections from the upper respiratory tract. As children grow up they tend to grow out of the problem, usually by the age of ten. Some people may have recurring bouts into childhood. Sufferers of glue ear may feel dizzy.

The symptoms of glue ear in children include;
- some children daydream and are inattentive at school
- some children speak too loudly; others talk less or mispronounce words
- some children fret because ear infections can cause discomfort or pain
- some children can be frustrated by not hearing properly and may be overactive or have temper tantrums
- some children may want the TV or video volume turned up or may not hear the door bell or a car parking outside the house.

Causes of Glue ear

Glue ear is also known as Otitis media with effusion, persistent middle - ear effusion or secretory Otitis media. This condition is due to a dysfunction of the Eustachian tube. The Eustachian tube links the tympanic cavity to the nasopharanyx, and the tube is the structure which brings air into the middle ear to keep it healthy and also act as a pressure regulating system so that the air pressure on each side of the ear drum is equal.

The tube is usually closed but opens for a fraction of a second about every three minutes in response to swallowing and yawning. If this opening action doesn't occur, a vacuum is formed. The middle ear lining becomes inflamed and a thin fluid leaks from it into the middle ear. The congested fluid thickens, causing glue ear.

The incidence of glue ear is affected by exposure to tobacco smoke and also factors such as brothers or sisters who may have had glue ear and the effects of allergens such as dust, house mites and animal fur.

Research in Newcastle, UK which has been supported by the charity Defeating Deafness (the Hearing Research Trust) has found that reflux of gastric juice (pepsin and acid) into the middle ear is a major cause of glue ear. Bacteria which should be consumed by the acid fluid of the stomach are regurgitated up into the oesophagus and then transported up and into the Eustachian tube via the upper respiratory tract. Drugs that reduce gastric juice production and prevent its reflux should help prevent glue ear occurring and recurring. This research also found that molecules which signal between cells (Cytokines) found in the 'glue' stimulate mucus production and stimulate the cells to further stimulate mucus secretion. Therefore, the disease persists because of the chronic stimulus for the cells to keep producing mucus, the major component of the effusion - drug treatments may be able to break this circle.

In Denmark, Bjørn Larsen an eminent reflexologist feels that milk and dairy products which cause allergic reactions and intolerance is a major cause of middle ear infections and that a removal of milk from the diet has led to a 50% reduction of symptoms in his patients. The processing and treatment of milk is the main reason for non-toleration and that those children who get the milk direct from the cow do not experience the same problems.

Dr Ulf Schønsted - Madsen also from Denmark thinks that children with different types of middle ear infection have either poor Eustachian tube function, frequent upper respiratory tract infections, exposure to environmental pollution such as smoking or a mainly milk diet with too little iron which leads to a weakening of the immune system.

The Ear Drum/Tympanic membrane

If the ear drum, which is a durable structure, is damaged, and is unable to vibrate properly it will not be able to transmit sound from the outer ear canal through to the ossicle bones, which are situated in the tympanic cavity behind the ear drum. The first of the ossicles, the hammer/malleus, is attached directly to the ear drum and its silhouette should be visible when the ear is examined medically with an otoscope.

The ear drum can be perforated ('burst') naturally in two ways;
O **traumatically** - by being exposed to a loud noise such as an explosion or by being damaged in an accident
O **pathologically** - by a change in atmospheric pressure which acts on the ear drum when there is an infection behind the membrane in the post tympanic cavity. It is for this reason that there are inherent risks when going diving or flying with an inner ear infection. When there is conductive deafness caused by a sudden pressure change in an aircraft or when diving this is known as barotrauma.

Cholesteatoma

This condition is caused when the outer part (Pars flaccida) of an ear drum does not heal completely after a perforation; skin cells and debris collect and infection arises which can spread from the ear drum to the mastoid process and then to the brain. **If this condition is not treated speedily it can become life threatening. It is vital for an ear drum to be checked by a medical practitioner to ensure that it has completely healed.**

The Ossicles

The three bones; the hammer/malleus, the anvil/incus and the stirrup/stapes are collectively known as the ossicles. Theiir function is to transmit sound across the middle ear through to the inner ear (labyrinth). The hammer is attached to the back of the ear drum, the stirrup to the inner ear and to each other by a system of ligaments. Two small muscles hold the chain rigid and they articulate with each other.

To work properly these bones should have no obstruction to their movement. As they are bones they are subject to conditions which affect other bones in the body for example Paget's Disease (the process of bone formation is disrupted especially in the middle aged and elderly), Osteogenesis imperfecta (a form of osteoporosis which leads to microscopic fractures in the stapes bone), osteoarthritis (wear and tear), tumours, autoimmune disorders such as rheumatoid arthritis and nutritional disorders which may all soften bones and cause them to lose their shape and motility.

Perhaps the most common condition is the disorder otosclerosis of the stapes bone (the smallest of 206 bones in the body) whereby the base of the stapes becomes a fixed overgrown spongy bone and so cannot move freely and intrinsically transmit sound to the inner ear.

Sensorineural (perceptive) deafness

Sensorineural deafness occurs only when there are problems in the inner ear, with the acoustic nerve connection to the brain and in the brain itself.

The Inner Ear

The part of the inner ear which deals with the hearing process is the cochlea. This is a closed tube wound 2.75 times and it resembles a snail's shell (hence the London Cockney slang term 'shelllike' when alluding to the ear). It is only 0.25 inches (0.6 cms) in length and height. As we saw in chapter 3 there are thousands of specialised cells, which resemble hairs when examined under a microscope lining the Organ of Corti (lamina spiralis) which is the basal layer of the inner membrane of the Cochlea.

There are two types of these hair cells on the organ of Corti; the inner cells and the outer cells. At birth we have about 35,000 hair cells; at the age of 18 we have approximately 15,000 outer and 5,000 inner hair cells. Although they reduce in efficiency with ageing, or through other reasons, their reduced efficiency does not automatically lead to deafness. With 15,000 hair cells there is still normal hearing and this state persists until a drop to 5 - 6,000; with 3,000 hair cells there are major problems and those people with 1,000 or less are likely to have congenital hearing loss or other long term hearing loss.

With ageing, cell depletion is concentrated at the narrowest (nearest) end, which is where the high frequency, shortest hair cells are located. This does not normally lead to a reduction in our ability to hear speech, because the human voice is generally at a lower pitch than this hearing range. Many animals, such as dogs, have a higher range of hearing than humans do and this is evidenced by the fact that they can hear special whistles which humans cannot hear. Humans are not able to replace hair cells which do not work. Birds, amphibians and fish on the other hand can regenerate their hair cells (source: 'Regeneration of Cochlear Hair Cells by Mark E. Warchol, PhD from Physiology of the Ear (2nd Edition) ed. Jahn ISBN. 1- 5659-3994-8) This age related degeneration is called presbyacusis and it is thought that 25% of the population in the UK need a hearing aid to cope with it.

The organ of Corti, and the tube in which it lies, is narrower at the proximal end (nearest the oval window), which is the junction with the middle ear. It is to this organ, that the hair cells are attached.
The hair cells have different lengths, and different positions within the cochlea; the short fibres are located in the first part of the cochlea, the medium fibres in the centre and the long fibres at the end of the cochlea (nearest the round window);
Outer hair cells
short length fibres - high frequency (20,000 to 1500 cycles per second (cps; measured in hertz (Hz))
medium length fibres - medium frequency (1500 - 500 cps)
Inner hair cells
long length fibres - low frequency (500 to 20 cps).

The different frequencies of vibration (the tones of sound) cause hair cells in the different parts of the cochlea to vibrate; for instance, if it is a high pitched sound which is being heard, the short hair cells will be vibrated. The cochlea, like the rest of the inner ear labyrinth, contains two distinct fluids, which are separated by a membrane. The outer fluid is called perilymph and the inner fluid is called endolymph. While the fluid has a watery appearance the perilymph has a main constituent of potassium (K) and the endolymph has a main constituent of sodium (Na). These elements should be in balance and any imbalances can be detected by urea and electrolyte tests.
The fluid is moved by the action of the stapes bone, which works as a piston on the outer side of the labyrinth to which it is attached and the vibration is transmitted through to the fluid. While, generally, problems in the inner ear are regarded as sensorineural, if the stirrup bone does not work properly it will not do its work efficiently. The inner ear fluid consequently is not being moved as it should - this could therefore be regarded as a cause of conductive hearing loss.

There are other reasons why the cochlea hair cells are damaged, and these include;
- ☐ if a mother has rubella (German measles) while she is pregnant this may adversely affect the cochlea of the baby. This is a rare occurrence with approximately 1 in 1000 babies being born deaf
- ☐ if severe jaundice is contracted soon after birth
- ☐ if a disease, such as mumps or meningitis is contracted
- ☐ if there is an adverse reaction to certain drugs such as streptomycin
- ☐ if a specific viral infection is present in the inner ear/labyrinth
- ☐ if Ménière's disease is contracted
- ☐ if there is exposure to loud noise for a long time. Under employment legislation, if a worker is in danger suitable ear protection in the form of ear protectors or ear plugs must be made available
- ☐ if there is a serious head injury with a skull fracture.

The Auditory/Acoustic/Cochlear nerve

The auditory nerve is the part of the vestibulocochlear nerve related to hearing and is the cranial nerve linking the inner ear to the brain.

A rare, benign tumour (an acoustic neuroma) can arise from the supporting cells that surround the nerve usually in the internal auditory meatus, which is the canal in the skull through which the nerve passes. Its growth rate is approximately 1mm each year. These neuromas are about 5- 7% of primary range brain tumours and there are a few hundred cases every year in the United Kingdom. They most commonly occur in people between the ages of 40 -60. More women are affected than men.

The cause of an acoustic neuroma is unknown; sometimes the nerves on both sides of the head are affected simultaneously and could be part of a widespread neurofibromatosis, a disease which brings changes in the skin and bones as well as the nervous system.

As well as causing deafness an acoustic neuroma can cause tinnitus (noises in the ear), intermittent hearing loss, loss of balance, dizziness or pain in the affected ear. As a tumour gets bigger it may compress the brain stem and cerebellum so causing ataxia (loss of coordination). As it expands, a tumour presses either on the Trigeminal nerve, which runs through the tympanic cavity causing pain or on the abducent cranial nerve causing double vision.

With a large tumour, which may impinge on any one of a number of cranial nerves, other symptoms may be - loss of taste to anterior tongue, difficulty to close lower eyelid, facial weakness, hoarseness or difficulty in chewing.

Diagnosis of the condition is made by hearing tests and tests of balance, such as the caloric test or electronystagmography test followed up by x-rays, CT (computed tomography) scanning or MRI (magnetic resonance imaging) tests which visualise the condition of the internal auditory meatus. Treatment is by surgery and whilst there is normally no residual damage to the acoustic nerve and hearing, occasionally numbness to part of the face can come from unavoidable damage to neighbouring nerves, which may occur during the operation.

Another problem can be hereditary nerve deafness; this is a genetic disorder and can affect sufferers either from birth or in later life. Whilst this condition can be a severe handicap many can overcome it as is the case of a brilliant young English female opera singing star. To allow her to perform she wears analogue in-the-ear hearing aids.

The Brain

There are a number of brain disorders which can impair the function of the whole brain which in turn reduces the quality of hearing. It has to be remembered that brain cells destroyed through injury or disease cannot be replaced so again function of all senses, including hearing, may be affected.

The efficiency of the brain can be affected by some or a combination of the following;
- ☐ Impaired blood and oxygen supply
- ☐ injury
- ☐ infection within the brain
- ☐ tumours - such as acoustic neuromas
- ☐ degeneration
- ☐ other disorders - which are characterised by their symptoms rather than their cause; migraines for example.

The practicalities of hearing and ear testing

We have already discussed the mechanics (physiology) of the transmission of sound within the ear and how it is transformed to nerve impulses which travel to the brain for processing and the differences between conductive and sensorineural deafness/ hearing impairment. It will be useful at this point to outline what hearing is and how it can be tested. The results of testing would indicate the cause of deafness and from this the correct treatment should follow.

The source of external noise

The outer ear (pinna/auricle), with its basic shape, is designed to channel external sounds into the ear canal. Information is needed from both ears to determine the direction from which different sounds are coming. The difference in time taken for any sound to reach the ears and the comparative difference in volume are the factors used by the brain to calculate the exact position of the source(s) of the noise.

Testing the ears

The consultation

The only parts of the ear which can be examined physically by a medical practitioner are the pinna, the ear canal and the ear drum. This examination is done with the use of an otoscope/auriscope. Before any examination is made the patient should be asked a number of questions such as;

- the nature of the problem
- how the problem affects you
- whether one or both ears are affected
- whether there is a history of ear problems in you or your family
- what your lifestyle is.

These questions form a questionnaire or case history and they should remain confidential. If a complementary therapist, who should be qualified and insured, such as an ear candling therapist, is going to carry out a treatment a similar consultation/ case history should be compiled.

Visually checking the external ear, ear canal and ear drum

After taking the consultation/case study the practitioner will examine the external ear (pinna) and test for tenderness behind it. This will indicate if there is inflammation in the middle ear or boils/swollen glands around the ear and neck; other conditions such as melanomas will also be apparent. The ear canal is then checked with an otoscope for wax, foreign bodies or any unhealthy discharge (a symptom of Otitis externa). Damage to the ear canal due to the patient pushing items, such as baby cotton buds, into the canal will also be seen. This damage, or the result of conditions such as eczema or psoriasis in the ear canal, may be the cause of itching (pruritus).

The practitioner will also use the otoscope to examine the ear drum to see if it is intact, and whether the tympanic cavity, which lies behind the ear drum is clear of infection. The silhouette of the hammer bone, which is attached to the ear drum, should be visible behind the ear drum in a healthy middle ear. If it is thought that the ear drum is perforated this can be confirmed by using a pneumatic attachment to the otoscope. If the ear drum moves on compressing the attachment the membrane is intact, if there is no movement the membrane is perforated.

The Eustachian tube can be checked by asking the patient to close the nose and mouth and blow - pressure inside the head is increased and the ear drum bulges outwards. Swallowing then follows which normalises the pressure in the middle ear so pulling the ear drum back in again.

Using a tuning fork to decide whether hearing loss is conductive or sensorineural

Patients who suffer hearing loss can be tested by a doctor in several ways with a tuning fork. There are a number of tests - Weber, Chimani-Moos, Gelle, Bing and Modified Schwabach (absolute bone conduction) but the most common is the Rinne test. The Rinne test, which decides whether the loss is conductive or sensorineural, essentially compares the auditory acuity (sharpness) of each ear to bone and air conduction and is in three parts;

- Firstly - the fork, which most commonly has a frequency of 512 Hz, is struck gently on the hand bone of the doctor and then held against points on the midline of the skull of the patient, normally the forehead. The note of the higher frequency forks tends to decay quickly allowing insufficient time for the test to be carried out. Lower frequency forks tend to enhance perception by vibration sensation.

The patient will be asked whether they hear the sound equally, in both ears or more on one side, if there is a worse problem with one ear, the side which hears more clearly can give an indication of the type of deafness. If the sound is clearer in the better ear, deafness is likely to be sensorineural; if it is clearer in the worst ear it is more likely to be conductive. Where both ears are affected equally or components of both forms of deafness are suspected this test can be relatively inconclusive

☐ secondly - the tuning fork is held against the base of the skull and then moved to the ear to see whether you can hear it more clearly by bone conduction (against the skull) or by air conduction (at the ear hole). If the hearing is better through bone conduction, conductive deafness is indicated

☐ thirdly - the fork is held against the skull again with an ear blocked. If the ear canal is blocked the cochlea in the inner ear normally gets stronger signals from bone vibration than when it is not blocked. If the tone is heard more clearly when the canal is blocked this indicates either normal hearing or sensorineural deafness. The doctor will be aware of the volume of the tuning fork, so if it is unheard by the patient when the doctor can hear it this is strong evidence of deafness.

The test in its entirety will normally conclusively indicate whether hearing loss is conductive or sensorineural. The practitioner will then refer the patient to a specialist for other tests, depending on symptoms and responses to the tuning fork test and background knowledge in the case study and experience built up over many years examining ear problems. For example, if there is tinnitus in one ear this is an indication, to a doctor, of a possible benign cancer on the vestibulocochlear nerve.

Specialist testing

If a doctor feels it appropriate he will refer a patient to a specialist Ear, Nose and Throat (ENT) department, usually situated in a hospital. There are a number of tests which are available for hearing problems; there are other tests available for balance, motion and other conditions.

CT and MRI Scans

Scans

Scans are usually carried out if conductive hearing problems are indicated or if a vestibulocochlear nerve tumour is possible. The result of the scan will indicate to the doctor whether the three ossicle bones are in correct alignment and so working properly and if the presence of a cancerous tumour can be discounted.

Audiometric testing and analysis

Audiometric testing and analysis is a complex technique used to measure the ear's responses to various sounds and patterns. An audiogram, which is a hearing response table, gives an accurate measurement of someone's hearing. Audiometry allows an analysis of someone's ability to perceive different pitches and volumes of sound.

Testing is usually carried out inside a soundproof compartment by a technician, who is outside visible through a small window. The patient will normally be wearing a large pair of headphones to isolate him/her even more.

If one ear is worse than the other, it is usual to test the good ear first and then play 'white noise' into the good ear while the poor ear is being tested to stop the sound being conducted through from the good ear via the skull bones.

It is through the bones of the skull that the sound of one's own voice is resonated.

A range of pitches is played in one ear, then the other, with the volume starting at a very low level and then gradually increased. Most people's hearing responds most to sounds at a pitch of around 1000 Hz and it is at this level that most audiometric tests begin. Pitches are the then increased until the patient cannot hear the tone, frequencies are doubled each time and the patient presses a button each time they can hear the sound.

At each frequency the technician plays the sound starting at 0dB and increases in 5db steps until the sound is heard. The technician will then adjust the level until the patient can no longer hear the sound. The procedure will be the same in the second ear.

Sometimes, a second test will be carried out using a bone conduction microphone instead of headphones.

The most important range of hearing is between 500 and 2000 hertz with most speech occurring within this range, as do sounds of telephones, alarm clocks, car horns and other things we need to listen to regularly. Most hearing loss occurs above this range, and as the hair cell loss from the organ of Corti is at the higher end of the range we rarely notice the effects of their damage and loss.

In the frequencies of sound most relevant to people, the level of volume reduction is important;

☐   a loss of up to 30 dB should be of little consequence - a person suffering at this level will be slightly hard of hearing

☐   a loss of up to 40 dB will mean that an individual might experience problems in group conversation or noisy parties

☐   a loss of 50 dB, such as could be experienced with a severe case of glue ear, would lead to the category of being a ' bit deaf"

☐   a loss of 60dB would mean difficulty with a telephone conversation

☐   a loss of 90dB would mean a sufferer is totally deaf to speech - being 'stone deaf'

Standard audiometric analysis is an excellent diagnostic tool but it has two drawbacks;

☐   pure tone does not replicate sound as heard in normal life and the brain can overcompensate for the loss in perceived volume (by a process called 'recruitment'). If recruitment occurs, a small increase in volume is heard as a much greater increase by the patient. This situation is also applicable to sufferers of tinnitus

☐   often patients can be slow, nervous, hesitant or express other traits which could lead to the recording button been pressed at the wrong time with incorrect values being deduced.

To eliminate these problems another technique called impedance audiometry, which uses a probe in the ear, can be used. This gives an accurate result.

By using audiometric analysis, a specialist can usually make a diagnosis of the cause of hearing problems. A patient should ask the General Practitioner to be referred for this form of test to be carried out if he/she thinks that they suffer from deafness, hearing loss or tinnitus. The determination of the presence, or not, of a tumour is one of the most important emotional issues which can be resolved by this form of testing.

There are two other conditions, which should be examined when considering deafness and hearing impairment. These are;

☐ **Tinnitus**

☐ **Ménière's Disease**

Tinnitus

Tinnitus is one of the most common of the ear conditions and could be loosely defined as 'ringing in the ears'. It has been estimated that one in ten adults of the population of the United Kingdom suffers from the symptoms of the condition to different degrees (Royal National Institute for Deaf People fact sheet 'Questions about tinnitus'). It is more common in those people over forty years of age although all ages suffer from it including children. Tinnitus is more common in those with hearing loss but those without hearing loss can suffer from it and you can have hearing loss without suffering from the condition. Tinnitus originates from the Latin word 'tinnere' meaning 'to ring'.

The link between sensitivity and sound and tinnitus

About 40% of tinnitus sufferers are more sensitive than normal to common sounds. There are two types of sensitivity to sound;

● **hyperacusis** - everyday sounds are uncomfortable or painfully loud even when most other people are not bothered by them, this condition is also known as 'recruitment'

● **misophonia** - particular sounds are extremely irritating although there is no particular sensitivity to sounds in general. If the dislike is strong enough to be considered a phobia (a persistent and irrational fear of, and desire to avoid, a particular object or situation) then the term **phonophobia** is used.

Tinnitus has two major categories; **objective and subjective tinnitus**. Subjective tinnitus is much more common than objective tinnitus.

Objective tinnitus

This form of tinnitus appears as a bodily noise in the ear area. A doctor can hear it through the stethoscope; some cases of constant pitched tinnitus can only be heard with an implanted microphone and an amplifier. There is no hearing defect as such, because noise really exists. There are only a few problems that can be the cause of objective tinnitus;

☐ the wearing of the jaw (TMJ) joint gives a roughness, which causes a noise to be made when the bones rub -the noise resembles grinding or growling

☐ the muscles in the roof of the mouth go into periodic spasm generating vibration in the skull - the noise will be a clicking or bumping

☐ the blood flow can be irregular in the ear region - the noise will be rhythmic, in time with the pulse and be pulsing, swishing or throbbing.

Although objective tinnitus can be diagnosed by the ENT specialist it is quite difficult for surgery to be helpful.

Subjective tinnitus

Subjective tinnitus is much more common than objective tinnitus and although the exact causes of it are uncertain, there are two main possibilities for the problem, these are;

☐ **malfunction of the cochlea**, particularly damage to the hair cells on the organ of Corti

☐ **disturbed nerve signal transmission** from the inner ear to the brain, for example tumour growth on the vestibulocochlear nerve.

The hearing part of the brain (the auditory cortex) which filters out sounds which are not important and filters in those which are important picks up the weak tinnitus signal which is generated by the inner ear and auditory nerve. If an individual is annoyed or anxious by the perception of the signal the sound response system will tune into the tinnitus and it will become more significant.

Other specific causes of tinnitus

Other causes of tinnitus are;

☐ **Ménière's Disease** - tinnitus associated with Ménière's Disease is normally low pitched like buzzing or a strong wind

☐ **reaction to certain drugs** - temporary tinnitus can be caused by aspirin, which can also induce temporary deafness, usually at a high dose; quinine and other anti-malaria drugs. Other drugs, which can have an ototoxic (poisonous) effect are a certain group of antibiotics known as aminoglycosides, including Streptomycin

☐ **some strong diuretics** (which are drugs designed to eliminate excess water from the body), also have ototoxic properties. There are other drugs and compounds, which may cause tinnitus and/or hearing loss; the doctor will be aware of the risks of prescribing these drugs and will take the risks into account. It is most important to discuss any prescription of drugs with the doctor, and not to stop taking any medication without telling him/her

☐ **phantom tinnitus** - if the acoustic nerve has been damaged and hearing loss happens it is possible for any surviving nerve tissue to spontaneously create phantom noise which the brain will then interpret as sound even if someone is deaf

☐ **head injury** - after an accident, which sets off tinnitus, a high-pitched whine can be experienced

☐ **catarrh** - a rare form of tinnitus is caused when the Eustachian tube becomes blocked with catarrh, so causing pressure problems in the middle ear. Normally, this form of tinnitus is temporary and fades when the tube becomes clear

☐ **exposure to loud noise** - loud or piercing noise sources are possible causes of tinnitus which can be temporary or permanent. It is more likely to occur if exposure is over a long period of time. These sources of noise can also cause temporary or permanent hearing loss, examples are;

- ☐ **loud discos and live music concerts** (rock, pop and classical music) at which audience and performers alike are at risk
- ☐ **aircraft noise** when taking off and landing
- ☐ **firearms shooting**
- ☐ **sirens and burglar alarms**
- ☐ **high pitched equipment** like dentist's drills and vehicle panel beating hammers
- ☐ **arteriosclerosis** - this has a strong effect on blood pressure, and hence tinnitus
- ☐ **tumour on the vestibulocochlear nerve** - these are usually benign and removable by surgery
- ☐ **excessive ear wax** in the outer ear canal pressing on the ear drum
- ☐ **problems with ear irrigation and cleansing.**

Research and tinnitus

Recent research findings in neurophysiological and neuro-imaging have established that persistent tinnitus involves changes in the body's central nervous system as well as problems with the hearing mechanism.

Research by a team led by Professor Carole Hackney at the University of Keele, UK which is supported by the charity Defeating Deafness (The Hearing Research Trust) is looking at how signals are carried from the ear along the auditory nerve to the brain. The chemicals responsible for transmitting signals along nerves are called neurotransmitters; one of these - glutamate - is active in the inner ear and its connections with the acoustic nerve. There is an identified 'transporter' molecule GLAST (which is normally found in the brain) which removes glutamate, excessive amounts of which cause damage to the surrounding cells. It is possible that a failure of the 'mop up' system could result in inappropriate levels of glutamate in the system, so causing tinnitus.

At the University of Regensburg, Germany early research has found that sufferers have increased biochemical activity in the region of the brain concerned with hearing. The activity was reduced by applying a source of magnetic stimulation to the head inducing an electric current in the brain - this promising long term research is ongoing. Research by Professor Edzard Ernst of Exeter University, England has indicated that using Ginkgo Biloba can improve micro circulation in the inner ear so helping tinnitus.

Triggers of tinnitus

The following things have been proposed as triggers, and not causes, of tinnitus, in many cases there is not enough evidence to back up assertions;
- ☐ **nicotine, caffeine and alcohol**
- ☐ **restricted classified drugs** such as cocaine and marijuana
- ☐ **excessive wax** in the ear canal and around the ear drum
- ☐ **ear irrigating** (previously syringing)
- ☐ **stress and anxiety.**

Many people experience two or more different noises at the same time, either continuously or intermittently with periods of silence in between.

A bizarre episode happened when one of the author's friends whilst running in the London Marathon, was exposed to several American-style marching bands beginning their loud repertoire with a shrill, high pitched note just as he was passing them. The result was that he had ringing in his ears for quite a while after the race!

Balance problems

How do we balance?

The ability to remain upright and be able to move without falling over is a complex process, which needs information from three sources which is supplied to the cerebellum part of the brain from which instructions are supplied to different muscles in the body to contract or relax to enable balance to be achieved.

The three sources are; the eyes; sensory receptors/propriceptors in the skin, muscles, ligaments and capsules of joints; and the vestibular system consisting of the vestibule (utricle and saccule) and the three semicircular canals, which are contained in the labyrinth/inner ear.

Receptors are stimulated mechanically and they signal the direction of action of the acceleration of gravity as well as accelerations associated with linear motion. Many of the sensory endings, especially those in the skin concerned with the sensation of touch and pressure adapt to changes very rapidly and are better at signalling a change in force rather than the steady state. These work with the specialised receptors in the inner ear which sense linear accelerations and complement the dynamic rather than the static response of the receptors.

The generally distributed mechano-receptors also provide essential information about the spatial relationship and movement of one part of the body to the other parts. So in the absence of vision the relative position of the limbs can be accurately gauged. This proprioceptive/kinaesthetic sense is achieved mainly by information signalled by receptors in the capsules of joints, although muscle spindles and other stretch receptors in the tendons also play a part in the process.

The kinaesthetic receptors play an important part in the perception of the body's orientation relative to the external references. While the vestibular part of the inner ear signals the angular movement and attitude of the head with respect to the gravitational vertical it is also necessary for the brain to be informed about the position of the head on the trunk and of the limbs in relation to the trunk so that an adequate perception of the spatial orientation of the body and its appendages can be built up.

The cutaneous receptors in and below the skin which respond to pressure and touch are also important in that they allow a person to know what he/she is in contact with and this may influence movement and the reasoning behind movement of the body.

The eyes give the visual information about the body's position in relation to its surroundings. The sensory receptors give information about the position and movement of the various parts of the body and the vestibule and semicircular canals detect the direction and speed of head movements.

As normal body position results from neural input from the sources described above if hypofunction of one input happens then compensation by others usually takes place. Different tests are available to clinicians and these include;

- Romberg's test
- Unterberger's test
- Gait test
- Fitzgerald-Hallpike bithermal caloric test (which stimulates and records eye nystagmus (continual oscillation of eyeballs)
- Electronystagmography - recording eye movements electrically.

Disorders which affect balance

There are a number of disorders which affect the middle and inner ear which in turn affect balance including;

☐ **Labyrinthitis** which is a viral or bacterial inflammation of the labyrinth/inner ear

☐ **Ménière's disease** which is thought to be an abnormally high pressure of the fluid in the vestibular part of the labyrinth

☐ **Otitis media**, which is inflammation of the middle ear, can affect the inner ear as well with a resultant loss of balance.

These ear disorders can often cause dizziness or vertigo and impaired hearing.

The sensory nerve pathways in the spinal cord which carry information from the proprioceptors may be damaged as a result of spinal tumours, disorders of the circulation or a deficiency of vitamin B.12.

A tumour or stroke affects the cerebellum part of the brain and lead to jerkiness of limbs as well as possible speech disorders and general impaired muscle coordination.

Dizziness and vertigo

Dizziness and vertigo are symptoms of many differing conditions with varying degrees of seriousness and should be considered separately.

Dizziness

This is a sensation of imbalance and light-headedness. It may be a mild brief symptom that occurs on its own or it may be part of a more prolonged serious attack of vertigo. Attacks are caused by a momentary fall in the pressure of blood reaching the brain, for example when getting up quickly from a sitting or lying position (this is why therapists must take care when a client arises from a massage couch) - this phenomenon is called postural hypotension (PH). PH is a condition more common in the elderly or in people taking antihypertensive drugs whose aim is to treat high blood pressure. Similar symptoms may come from a temporary, partial blockage in the arteries that supply the brain - the transient ischaemic attack, which are the symptoms of a stroke lasting less than 24 hours.

There are many **other causes of dizziness**, including;

☐ **tiredness**

☐ **stress**

- ☐ anaemia
- ☐ **hypoglycaemia** - low blood sugar level, which is especially relevant to diabetics
- ☐ **Glue ear and other middle ear infections**
- ☐ **labyrinthitis** - infection of the inner ear balance organs
- ☐ **eye strain**
- ☐ **wearing bifocal or veriflex glasses**
- ☐ **brain tumour**
- ☐ **side effects from prescribed drugs that affect circulation** e.g. for high or low blood pressure
- **heart attack**
- ☐ **Alzheimer's disease**
- ☐ **subdural haemorrhage** - bleeding between the outer two membranes that cover the brain
- ☐ **brain disease.**

Vertigo

Vertigo is different to dizziness or faintness in that the sufferer has an illusion either that he/she is spinning in relation to the surroundings or the surroundings are spinning in relation to him/her. The spinning sensation is either horizontal or vertical.

When vertigo is severe it is often accompanied by nausea, vomiting and even collapse. Nystagmus (flickering of the eyelids) is an important indicator.

Vertigo is caused by disturbance in the vestibular part of the labyrinth/inner ear or in the vestibular part of the vestibulocochlear nerve, which goes to the brain from the inner ear.

Different conditions causing Vertigo

Although vertigo can be experienced by healthy people when going sailing or on amusement park rides it is normally a result of a specific condition which often leads to vomiting and unsteadiness. The conditions include;
- ☐ **Labyrinthitis** - viral or bacterial inflammation of the labyrinth/inner ear
- ☐ **Ménière's Disease** - when attacks can be severe enough to cause the sufferer to fall to the ground ('drop' or 'shove' attacks)
- ☐ **Cervical (neck area) osteoarthritis** - this is a degenerative (wear and tear) condition which affects the joints between the vertebrae. Elderly people are the main sufferers. Pain and stiffness can be exacerbated as a result of turning the head or moving the neck suddenly
- ☐ **Tumour of the brain stem**
- ☐ **Multiple Sclerosis** - a progressive disease of the central nervous system which is thought to be an autoimmune disorder
- ☐ **Acoustic neuroma** - which is an intracranial condition
- ☐ **Meningitis** - when the acoustic nerve is affected
- ☐ **Vertebrobasilar insufficiency** - narrowing of the blood vessels that supply part of the brain stem

- ☐ **Migraine** - that involves blood vessels in the brain stem
- ☐ **Alternobaric vertigo** - due to a sudden decrease as experienced when an aeroplane dives or when a deep sea diver rises too quickly to the surface. With divers there seems be an association with either difficulty in 'clearing' the ears, upper respiratory tract infection or being adventurous
- ☐ **Vertigo of childhood** - with vomiting, in ages one to five years
- ☐ **Gastric/stomachal vertigo**
- ☐ **Lateral vertigo** - usually suffered by occupants of cars and trains when watching the rapid passing of objects such as trees or posts
- ☐ **Horizontal vertigo** - usually occurs when lying flat
- ☐ **Objective vertigo** - a sensation that stationary objects are in motion
- ☐ **Ocular vertigo** - caused by a dysfunction of the eye(s)
- ☐ **Post-traumatic vertigo** - following a concussive head injury, this is self limiting
- ☐ **Toxic vertigo** - due to toxic effects of drugs or to metabolic disorders
- ☐ **Apoplectic vertigo** - sudden onset, possibly due to brainstem ischemia (insufficient supply of blood).

Often vertigo can be associated with other symptoms. Ménière's disease sufferers can also experience severe vomiting, tinnitus, nystagamus and hearing loss.

Vertigo may also be psychological in origin; if this is the case it is usually associated with agoraphobia (fear of open spaces).

A sensation of falling or looking down from a high place or looking up towards a height or a fear of heights is not a true form of vertigo.

Benign Paroxysmal Positional Vertigo (BPPV)

BPPV is the most common form of vertigo and BPPV means;
- ● **B**enign - it is not due to a serious disease (it can be disabling however)
- ● **P**aroxysmal - its duration is short (usually 5-30 seconds but sometimes up to two minutes)
- ● **P**ositional - it is caused by specific movement to and from certain postions; it is generally rotational and is different from spontaneous vertigo which is a symptom of Ménière's Disease, or movement - provoked which can be initiated by any movement
- ● **V**ertigo - an illusion of movement either of the sufferer or of the surroundings.

BPPV is thought to affect half the population at some time; it is rare in children and teenagers but accounts for half the vertigo cases in the over eighties. It may occur daily for years on end or recur in bouts lasting days or weeks.

The main movements which provoke BPPV are;
- ● lying flat
- ● sitting up from lying flat
- ● turning over in bed
- ● looking up
- ● bending down and looking to the side.

BPPV is caused by a transfer of fragments of microscopic chalk crystals from the vestibule to any one of the three semicircular canals (which are responsible for sensing rotation in the different planes). The fragments can be loosened by;
- any ear disease including a viral infection (vestibular neuritis)
- Ménière's Disease
- a head injury
- degeneration of the inner ear in old age
- no obvious cause.

Testing for BPPV

When attacks are not happening diagnosis is made from the patient's history together with excluding other conditions and disorders which can cause similar dizzy conditions. When attacks are occurring the Hallpike positional test is used for diagnosis. A patient will be sat on an examination couch and the body and head moved rapidly into different positions. If the test is positive the patient will become dizzy and nystagmus (repetitive eye movement) will occur. From the pattern of nystagmus a doctor can decide which canal and which ear is affected. Upon sitting up, vertigo will be repeated and the nystagmus will reverse. The test is repeated with the head turned the other way. The Hallpike test is positive (induces vertigo and nystagmus) when the affected ear is downward. Bilateral problems are up to 10% of cases. Other symptoms are positively ruled out.

Mal de debarquement syndrome (MDD)

Thankfully, this is a very rare condition, which mimics the sensation of getting off a boat and which occurs when there is prolonged exposure to motion which causes a brain imbalance. Astronauts can suffer from it when they land back on earth. This can be a longstanding condition; it is reported that one lady in England has suffered from the symptoms for over two years, and the treatment is to do rebalancing exercises - in short or long bursts, up to several hours at a time.

Ménière's Disease

A French physician called Prosper Ménière (1799 - 1862) first described the disease in 1861. Other medical conditions are often ascribed to the name of the practitioner who first wrote up the condition such as 'Bells palsy', which was first described by a Scottish physician, Dr Bell (b 1774).

Because of the number of conditions which make up the spectrum of Ménière's Disease some people prefer to use the term Ménière's Syndrome. Another description is Endolymphatic hydrops (an abnormal accumulation of fluid in body tissues or a sac) which does accurately describe the pathological findings of the condition.

Causes of Ménière's Disease

The Disease is thought to be caused by excessive endolymph fluid in the membranous labyrinth of the inner ear (especially the vestibule which affects balance), which causes dilation and increased pressure within the labyrinth, which can damage all of its parts including the adjacent cochlea. The cause of the changes could be an autoimmune factor - an abnormal reaction to tissue which has probably been altered by a virus.

A full blown condition affects 1 per 2,000-20,000 of the UK population (source: Ménière's Society Spin magazine No. 53) and it is more common in men than women. It is usually a late onset disease affecting predominantly Caucasian/Eurasian peoples. The racial distribution and familial clustering (7% in the UK) is strong evidence of genetic predisposition.

Some patients suffer from all symptoms of the Disease, while others may only suffer from some of the symptoms. It is a progressive disease which may affect one ear or both ears. Attacks can be incapacitating in the work, home and leisure environments.

Symptoms of Ménière's Disease

This inner ear disorder is characterised by recurring symptoms such as;
● **rotational vertigo**
● **roaring tinnitus**
● **nausea**
● **vomiting**
● **sweating**
● **visual disturbances**
● **violent headaches**
● **fluctuating hearing loss**
● **feeling of pressure ('fullness') in the affected ear(s)**
● **'shove' attacks and 'drop' attacks**
● **sinusitis and allergic rhinitus**

Attacks of vertigo can last from a few minutes to several hours. There can also be a feeling of pressure ('fullness') in the affected ear, both before and during the time of an attack. When there are large weather barometric pressure changes these can affect sufferers greatly.

Tinnitus and deafness can continue between attacks. Some people have clusters of attacks followed by periods of remission; others many have attacks with a long period, perhaps a year, in between.

Initially, the effects of the Disease are usually unilateral; both ears are often affected later. Unfortunately, as the disease progresses, hearing loss becomes more pronounced; attacks of vertigo on the other hand usually decrease in severity.

'Shove' attacks are spontaneous and happen without warning and are caused by a contraction of a muscle on the side of the body which forces a person in that direction. 'Drop' attacks (Tumarkin's Otolithic Crisis) are experienced in 1%-3% of sufferers and there is no loss of consciousness. A 'drop attack' is thought to be caused when a build up of pressure in the endolymphatic system bursts and the vestibular system (eyes, labyrinth and proprioceptive nerve endings) is overwhelmed; all the reflexes in the joints and muscle tone are lost and a person falls down.

Testing for Ménière's Disease

Because the symptoms of Ménière's disease are very similar to other hearing and balance problems there are a number of tests which can be carried out to diagnose the condition. These tests include a pure tone audiometry/hearing test, the caloric test and other specific tests; these tests are carried out in the ENT Department in a hospital.

The function of the balance mechanism of the vestibule/semicircular canals in the inner ear is tested by observing nystagamus/jerky eye movements when the head is placed in different positions or the whole body is turned and the outer ear is flooded, using a syringe, with water above and below body temperature (a caloric test). The flooding stimulates convection currents in the canals.

The reflex flickering of the eyes is either observed or electrically recorded (electronystagmography). If the labyrinth is normal, the flickering lasts for a predictable time. If the labyrinth is diseased, flickering will either not happen or finishes sooner than normal.

Other possible tests include;
- Tympanometry - which measures how well the Eustachian tube is working
- Speech audiometry - is a measure of the ability to understand speech
- Electronystagmography - measures the relation of the eyes to the brain and the possible cause of dizziness
- Posturography - this is a computerised test of balance which examines the co-ordination of the three inputs of balance; balance organs, eyes and joints
- Radiology - using an MRI scanner, a cross section picture of the inner head is built up and abnormalities such as tumours will be seen
- Glycerol dehydration - this test is unpleasant and its results are not conclusive
- Electrocochleography - is an electrical test of the cochlea organ of hearing.

Flying and Diving Ear and Paranasal Pressure Problems

There are a number of gas-filled cavities within the body. These are linked to the outside environment and it is important for them to be in equilibrium with the surrounding areas otherwise there will be adverse effects. The gas containing cavities are either semi-closed or closed; the ears, paranasal sinuses and lungs are semi-closed and the gastro-intestinal tract is closed.

Gas contained within the body is influenced by changes in the pressure outside the body i.e. as atmospheric pressure decreases (during ascent or on loss of cabin pressure, the volume of gas increases; during descent, the process is reversed and the volume of gas within the cavity decreases.

It would be expected that the degree of expansion of contained gas during change of atmospheric pressure would follow Boyle's law - 'The pressure of a given quantity of gas whose temperature remains unchanged varies inversely as its volume'. However, since the cavity walls are always moist, the gases contained within them are normally saturated with water vapour. If the volume of gas is increased by a reduction of pressure, the partial pressure of the water vapour will tend to fall; but the very rapid evaporation of the water from the lining film maintains full saturation under almost all conditions.

The partial pressure exerted by the water vapour is determined solely by temperature. It is normally 47 mmHg (at a temperature of 37 degrees C). For a given pressure ratio; the greater the altitude the greater the gas expansion, up to a limit of 63,000 feet when it is theoretically infinite. The process is self limiting because of increasing resistance of the surrounding tissue and gas expansion is therefore not infinite [Hg = mercury].

When there is unrestricted communication between a gas-filled cavity and the outside environment, such as in a properly functioning Eustachian tube, gas expansion occurs with little difficulty and no discomfort. If equilibrium is difficult to achieve e.g. when there is glue ear in the Eustachian tube the result will be pain and discomfort.

Effects on the Middle Ear

When Flying
When an aircraft takes off, the pressure of the air inside the middle ear and sinuses is the same as the airport's, often that of the pressure at sea level. As the aircraft climbs the cabin pressure falls to equate roughly to that found at around 9,000 feet which is the average height of a peak of a European mountain. If the fall is too great passengers would be starved of oxygen. The 9,000 feet level is a compromise between passenger safety and fuel costs. On descent the cabin air pressure rises.

The middle ear (post tympanic) cavity is separated from the outer ear canal by the tympanic membrane/ear drum. It is linked with the nasopharynx by the Eustachian tube whose upper (proximal) two thirds has soft walls which are normally collapsed. During ascent to altitude the gas in the cavity expands and the expanding gas escapes into the nasopharynx via the Eustachian tube. This equalises the pressure on either side of the ear drum.

Anatomically, the lower (pharyngeal) part of the tube acts as a 'one-way' valve and expanding air can escape into the atmosphere and the passive venting of the middle ear usually presents difficulties during decompression of gases. Intermittent passive ventilation during ascent is perceived as a 'popping' sensation as air escapes from the mouth of the tube into the pharynx. When ascending, the tube opens and gas escapes approximately once every 500 - 1,000 feet.

When descending, gas from the nasopharynx must enter the middle ear to maintain equilibrium between the atmospheric pressure outside and the gas pressure in the middle ear. Normally, the one-way valve mechanism of the Eustachian tube prevents the passive flow of gas back into the middle ear. The relative increase of pressure on the outer side of the tympanic membrane pushes the membrane into the middle ear cavity. As descent continues, the membrane is pushed further into the cavity unless gas can enter through the Eustachian tube. The distortion leads to a sensation of fullness in the ear and a decrease in hearing acuity (sharpness).

If descent continues further without pressure equalisation between the atmosphere and the middle ear the differential pressure across the ear drum causes pain. If an individual is susceptible a rapid change of pressure in the middle ear may also affect the vestibular balance organs of the inner ear with disorientation the result.

In order to equalise pressure across the tympanic membrane during descent it is usually necessary to carry out an active manoeuvre to open the Eustachian tube. This can be simply done by swallowing, yawning, jaw movements. It is for this purpose that passengers are given boiled sweets on aircraft. If these manoeuvres are not successful the nostrils have to be closed and pressure raised in the mouth and nose to be able to force gas into the cavity. This can be done by raising the floor of the mouth with the glottis shut. Alternatively, pressure in the lungs and respiratory tract can be raised by contracting expiratory muscles - Valsalva's manoeuvre. Trained aircrew can 'clear' ears every 1,000 to 4,000 feet. Swallowing can also cause contractions of the tiny muscles in the middle ear and movement of the ossicles which may be enough to transmit small pressure changes to the inner ear which may have significance for sufferers of conditions like Ménière's Disease.

Upper respiratory tract infection causes congestion and oedema of the mucosal lining of the Eustachian tube especially where it opens into the nasopharynx. The congestion can restrict gas entering the middle ear cavity during descent. The tympanic membrane will then be driven into the middle ear causing pain and deafness. If the situation continues the badly distorted ear drum will perforate/rupture with immediate pain relief.

The change in the tympanic membrane and middle ear produced by failure of adequate ventilation of the middle ear during descent is called otitic barotrauma. While it is usually associated with upper respiratory tract infection it can also be caused by too rapid descent or inadequate knowledge of the correct ways for ventilating the middle ear.

As a protection, an aircrew's helmet is in two parts - the skull and the ear muffs.

When Diving

The theory of the effects on the middle ear cavity and tympanic membrane of changes in pressure of gas are just as valid when someone goes diving as when he/she flies except that the steeper pressure gradient makes the problem more acute.

It is often necessary to hold the nostrils closed when jumping into the water from the side of a dive boat or pier. Not only will this protect the ear drum from damage but also reduce the likelihood of contaminated water being forced into the sinuses through the nose.

If there are excessive pressure fluctuations in the inner ear with movement of the ossicles being violent, pressure within the cochlea will cause it to burst in the vicinity of the round window. While this is a protective mechanism the loss of fluid will lead to persistent vertigo which may take weeks to clear unless surgical repair is undertaken.

It is important not to dive if there is any upper respiratory tract infection or Eustachian tube blockage as this will prevent correct equalisation of pressure either side of the membrane even in the first few feet of depth. The ears have to be 'cleared' correctly to ensure adequate ventilation of the middle ear cavity and the failure to achieve this can lead to pain and discomfort with a perforated ear drum being the most dramatic result.

In some divers who have not been able to 'clear' ears properly there is evidence of an inflamed ear behind which there is a haemorrhage into the middle ear.

It is advisable that anyone wanting to dive should check that both Eustachian tubes will clear freely with pressure changes. It is not recommended that 'clearing' take place repeatedly in a shallow depth as excessive force may cause some reactive swelling around the Eustachian tube meatus which does block and the dive has to be aborted.

That great care has to exercised when ascending from depth is well illustrated by the fact that Mark Ellyatt, a British scuba diver, descended 313 metres on 20 December 2003 in a twelve minute dive off Phuket, Southern Thailand to break the world depth record. His ascent took six hours forty minutes. Primarily he was protecting against the condition known as the 'bends' but he was also protecting his ears.

Colds and catarrh are more prevalent during the winter and this causes most loss of diving time. Intranasal decongestant drops/sprays or oral antihistamines can be taken.

When the ear has been damaged e.g. ear drum perforation the condition should be allowed to recover completely before diving again. Medical advice should be sought.

Excessive ear wax should be removed from the outer ear canal and no ear plugs or defenders worn as they may be forced into the ear under pressure so causing more damage.

In parts of the world, particularly the tropics, sand or coral may enter and damage the outer ear canal. Infection may arise and this should be treated medically and not by poking the canal with a sandy finger or baby bud!

'Reversed Ears'

This condition occurs when a diver wears a tight fitting rubber hood or cap and air may be trapped in the outer ear canal. Rising water pressure presses the covering tightly against the ear and the contained air volume can shrink no more. The Eustachian tube will open and the result is that the air pressure in the outer ear is increasingly lower than that of the surrounding tissues and middle ear. This is similar to attaching a suction pump to the ear and the ear drum will bulge outwards. While pain is not normally a feature of the condition there will be swelling and blistering of the canal wall.

The 'Reversed Ears' condition can be avoided if care is taken to ensure there is no barrier to pressure equalisation between the external ear and the surrounding water or if an overall hood is worn with connection between the ear and the nasopharynx.

Effects on the Paranasal Sinuses

The paranasal sinuses are cavities located in the bones of the face and skull. The frontal sinuses are linked to the nose by a relatively long duct while of each of the other sinuses - maxillary, ethmoidal and sphenoidal are connected to, and drain into the nose by a hole in its wall. The channels allow equilibrium to be established between them and the rest of the respiratory system.

During ascent and descent, when flying or diving, expanding and contracting gas contained within the sinus is linked with the gas in the nose and pressure is equal between both structures. If the mucous membrane lining the passage linking any sinus to the nose becomes inflamed and oedematous (swollen) normal passive ventilation of the sinus may be obstructed particularly during descent. Such a failure causes severe pain in any, or all of the cheeks, forehead or behind the nose possibly accompanied with watering of the eyes. Damage to the mucosal lining may happen with subsequent bleeding into the sinus cavity; this condition is called sinus barotrauma. The pain usually causes the dive to be aborted.

Auto-inflation of the sinus cavities is not easily achieved even by manoeuvres in which the pressure in the mouth and nose is raised above that of the environment. Nasal decongestants can be used.

Patulous (open) Eustachian Tube (PET)

Patulous Eustachian Tube is an annoying, benign condition whereby the Eustachian tube stays abnormally patent (open) instead of remaining closed for most of the time. The condition was first noticed by Schwartze in 1864 who noted a scarred atrophic ear drum moving simultaneously with respiration and then fully described by Jago in 1867 who had a patulous tube.

Causes of PET

The condition is more common in women than men and it occurs usually in adolescents and adults; rarely in children. It is usually brought about by another cause (idiopathically). These include;
- weight loss (sometimes caused by a chronic illness)
- pregnancy
- neurological disorders that may cause muscle atrophy e.g. stroke, multiple sclerosis and motor neurone disease
- adhesions forming in the nasopharynx following adenoidectomy or radiotherapy
- damage to the tensor veli palatini muscle after cleft palate surgery
- medication - oral contraceptives, diuretics
- fatigue
- stress or anxiety
- exercise
- Temporomandibular (TMJ) joint syndrome.

Normally, the tube is closed and only opens with swallowing or autoinflation. The closure is maintained by luminal (tube) and extraluminal (outside tube) factors. These factors include;
● 	intrinsic elasticity of the tube
● 	surface tension of the moist luminal surface
● 	extraluminal tissue pressure
● 	tone of the tensor veli palatine muscle dilates the lumen.

Pregnancy - alters opening pressures of the tube because of the change in surface tension
Weight loss - can be significant because of reduced tissue pressure and loss of fat deposits in the tube area
Oestrogens acting on the prostaglandin hormone affect surfactant (a wetting agent that reduces surface tension) production
Scarring in the postnasal space after adenoidectomy my lead to traction of the tube in the open position

Symptoms of PET
Many of the symptoms experienced by sufferers can be so great that as well as leading to a lack of sociability they can be psychologically damaging. The symptoms include;
● 	fluctuating aural fullness
● 	roaring tinnitus synchronous with nasal respiration
● 	audible respiratory sounds
● 	distorted autophony - the abnormal perception of one's own breath and voice sounds with echoing can be severe enough to interfere with speech production and a sensation of a 'plugged' ear - this is the most common symptom
● 	difficulty in eating because the noise of chewing is transmitted to the ear.

Vertigo and hearing loss can happen because a PET allows excessive pressure changes to occur in the middle ear- these pressure changes are then transmitted to the inner ear by ossicle bone movement. Symptoms may relate to cyclical changes occurring in the mucosa of the Eustachian tube; some sufferers may find relief from the associated mucosal congestion by lying down or putting the head between the knees. Compression of the jugular veins may also relieve symptoms but this procedure should be explained and demonstrated by an experienced medical practitioner before it is tried by a patient.
Patients can sniff repeatedly to close the tube but this may lead to long-term negative middle ear pressure. Decongestants or a ventilation tube/grommet can worsen symptoms.

Diagnosis of PET
While often PET is misdiagnosed because its symptoms appear the same as middle ear effusion, correct diagnosis can often be made on history alone. Full details of the conventional treatment of PET are included in chapter 7.

Degeneration
Elderley people can suffer from deafness/presbyacusis due to degeneration of the cochlea's hair cells; these cannot be regenerated as they can in birds, fish and reptiles.

Injury to the Ear
Repeated injuries to the pinna of the ear(s) of contact sports players such as boxers or rugby players can lead to the condition known as 'Cauliflower ear'. This occurs when there is a painful and swollen distortion of the ear flap (pinna) which has resulted from blows or friction that have caused bleeding within the soft cartilage structure.

Tumours
There are several types of tumour, which can affect the ear. Either a basal cell carcinoma (rodent ulcer) or a squamous cell carcinoma can affect the pinna. The squamous cell type may also affect the ear canal. Cancers of the middle and inner ears are rare. An acoustic nerve neuroma is benign and slow growing but because it can press on other parts of the ear it can cause deafness, imbalance or tinnitus (or a combination of these conditions).

Shingles
This is a common term for the viral infection herpes simplex. On the head this virus can be responsible for cold sores; conjunctivitis if it gets into the eye; and earache if it is herpes zoster opticus which can cause blisters in the outer ear canal.

Poisoning and Drugs
The labyrinth/inner ear is especially sensitive to damage by certain types of drug. The most important is the amino- glycoside antibiotics group including neomycin and gentamicin. These drugs can cause damage to the cochlea hair cells, especially if used in high concentration, particularly when there is kidney disease, which can delay the excretion of the drug from the body.Other drugs which can damage the ear include quinine, salicylates (including aspirin) and diuretic drugs frusemide, ethacrynic acid and bumetanide.If drugs are adversely affecting the ears it is said that the drugs have ototoxic properties. Aspirin should not usually be taken by children and adolescents under sixteen years of age.

Congenital ear defects which may affect a baby
There are several congenital defects which can affect a baby;
- [ ] absence or extreme narrowness of the external ear canal
- [ ] absence or distortion of the pinna (external ear flap)
- [ ] absence or deformity of the small ossicle bones of the middle ear
- [ ] hereditary (genetic) nerve deafness.

Goldenhar Syndrome
This extremely rare condition has different facial characteristics which can include being born with hearing loss, having ear tags or only one ear. This is associated with under development of the jaw and cheek on the same side of the face, if this is the only problem it is referred to as hemi-facial microsomia. If it is associated with other abnormalities, particularly of the vertebrae (hemi-vertebrae or under developed vertebrae usually in the neck) it is referred to as Goldenhar syndrome.
As well as hearing problems there may be heart problems, kidney abnormalities and other rarer congenital abnormalities. Many babies with the syndrome have poor weight gain in the first couple of years. Diagnosis is made clinically and no DNA abnormality has been identified. The risk of having another affected child is very small as it is almost a sporadic condition with only a few very rare familial cases. Plastic surgery can improve the growth of the face, particularly the jaw, by using bone distraction techniques to artificially lengthen the jaw bone. Children may need on-going orthodontic treatment. There are support groups in the UK and other countries.

CHAPTER 6: PREVENTION OF EAR PROBLEMS

Introduction

In the previous chapter we briefly touched on the importance of protecting the ears. The ears themselves contain a number of protective mechanisms. If people, especially those who are most at risk, take additional precautionary steps, then a number of ear problems, which have already developed can be minimised or eliminated completely. There are, however, a number of ear problems, which cannot be affected by any actions people can take.

There is an old adage 'that prevention is better than cure'. In the next chapter we will look at the different forms of treatment of ear problems which are available; both self-help and medical intervention. There is a certain amount of crossover between prevention and treatment of problems; one of the most obvious examples of this is the importance of dietary intake.

As we know, the ears have two functions; hearing and balance, we will look at hearing problems first; balance problems will follow and general ear conditions will conclude this chapter.

CONDUCTIVE HEARING LOSS

The outer ear canal

In the external curved ear canal (external auditory meatus), there can be blockages which are most commonly caused by excessive ear wax. While wax is necessary, as a protective, it should only be found in the outer third of the canal, which is the location of the wax producing glands. Problems arise when people try to clean their ear canals with an implement such as a cotton ear bud, plastic pen cap end, twisted cloth, toothpick or similar. The result usually is that the wax is pushed down the canal and can adhere to the ear drum, hence reducing the sound waves reaching it and/ or its motility with a subsequent hearing loss there is also the possibility of damage to the canal wall with the risk of infection.

GP practice nurses and doctors, who treat blocked ear canals can often recount lurid stories of other objects which they have found. These include small toys, coins, seeds - some of which are germinating in the warm and moist canal and insects (dead or alive).

Other debris, which can be found in the ear canal, includes dried soap, shaving foam and shampoo residue which has not been cleansed from the ears; sand granules, which stick in children's (and adults') ears when they are playing in the water or on the beach at the seaside on holiday. If people have trouble with their ears, which may itch (pruritus) they should consider inserting suitable earplugs when their ears may be in contact with water and using suitable eardrops such as olive oil to soothe the skin.

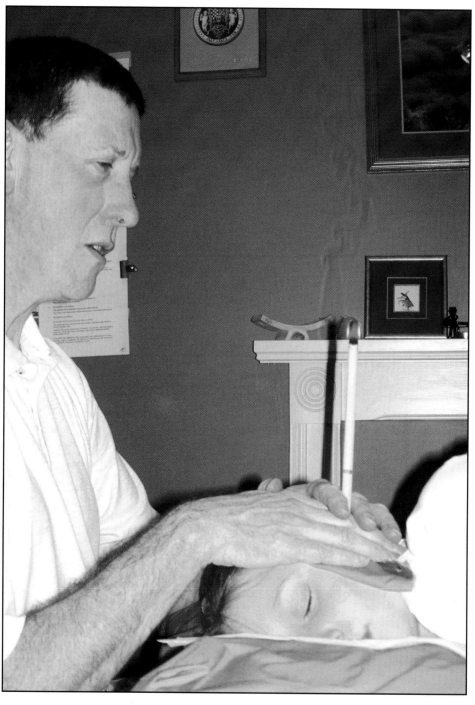

Author carrying out an ear candling treatment

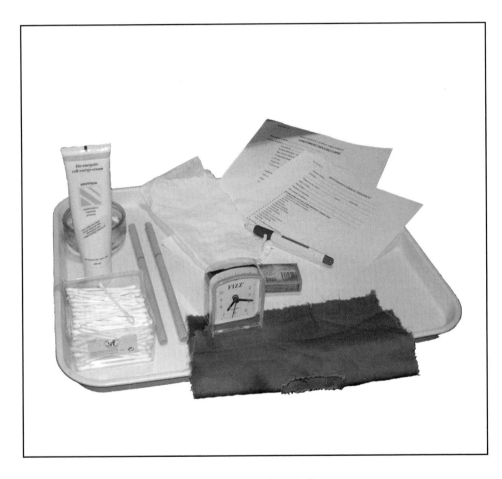

Equipment needed for an ear
candling treatment

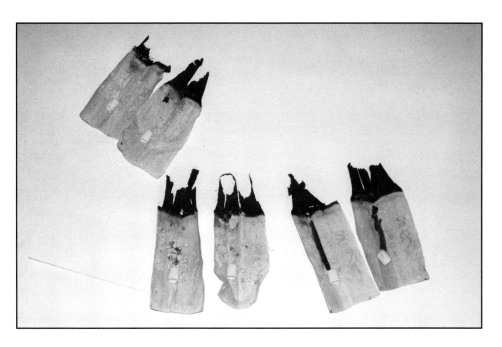

Different types of residue found in used ear candles

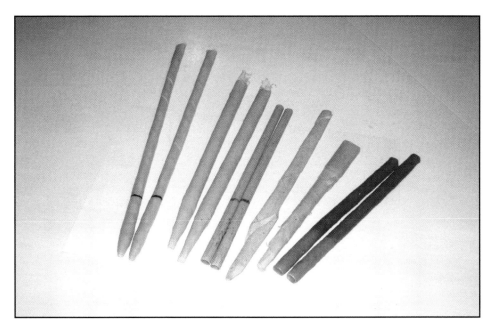

Examples of different types of ear candles

The Author's Right Ear
(auricle)

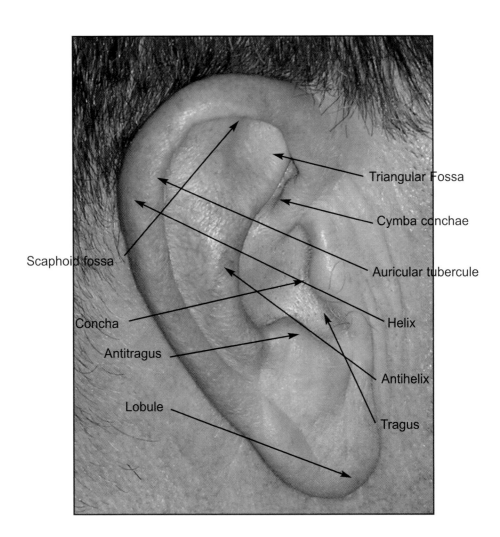

Triangular Fossa

Cymba conchae

Scaphoid fossa

Auricular tubercule

Concha

Helix

Antitragus

Antihelix

Lobule

Tragus

Parts of the ear (scale x 3)

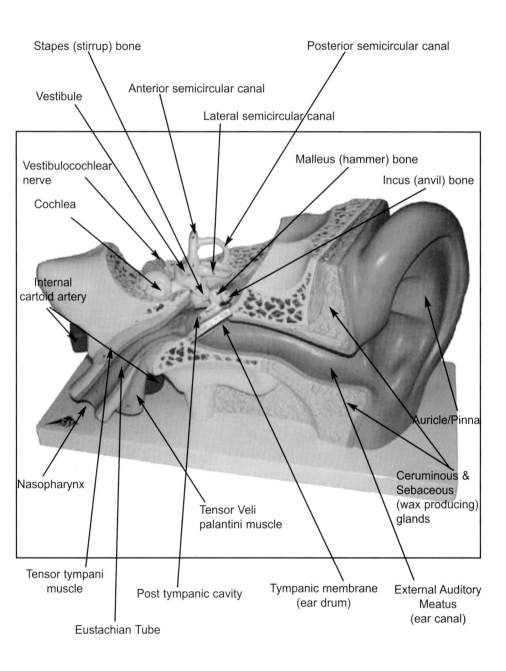

Stapes (stirrup) bone

Posterior semicircular canal

Vestibule

Anterior semicircular canal

Lateral semicircular canal

Vestibulocochlear nerve

Malleus (hammer) bone

Incus (anvil) bone

Cochlea

Internal cartoid artery

Auricle/Pinna

Nasopharynx

Ceruminous & Sebaceous (wax producing) glands

Tensor Veli palantini muscle

Tensor tympani muscle

Post tympanic cavity

Tympanic membrane (ear drum)

External Auditory Meatus (ear canal)

Eustachian Tube

Examples of hearing tests

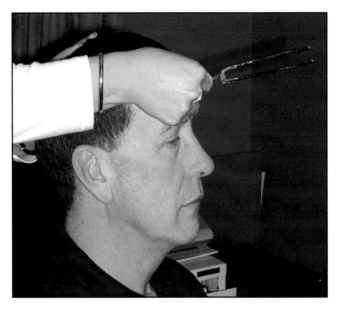

Weber test. The tuning fork is firmly placed on the forehead

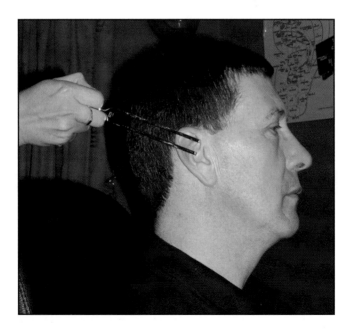

Rinne test. The tuning fork firmly on the mastoid bone

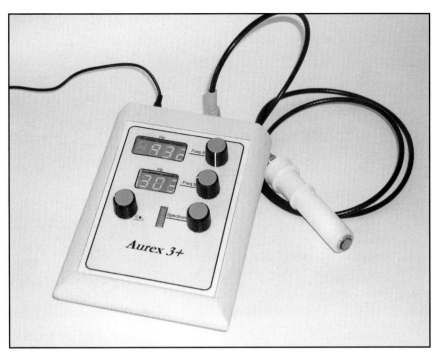

Aurex 3 plus Tinnitus therapy device
(picture courtesy of Shrewsbury Medical Ltd)

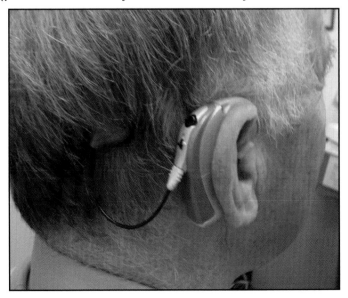

Example of a cochlear implant in place
(picture courtesy of Advanced Bionics)

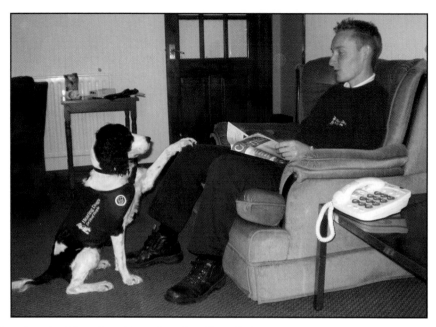

Samba (a Hearing Dog for the Deaf) is practicing her alert for the telephone with hearing dog trainer Ben Sargeant

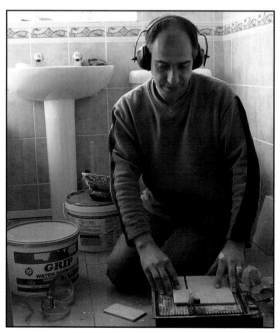

Ian Carley wearing appropriate ear protection doing DIY at home

People can be in either a noisy or dirty (or both) working or leisure environment. Whilst there is appropriate legislation to protect workers in the workplace very often unfortunately only the minimal protection in the way of earplugs or other ear defenders is offered. Many companies in the UK, such as Mars Foods in Slough, Bucks, where I worked doing seated massage during national Back Care week, offer their employees an excellent range of appropriate clean ear protectors, which are easily available throughout the production facility.

If the daily noise level is 85dB (A) or above the employer must inform workers of the risks and how the ears can be protected and provide ear protectors and maintain them in good repair. Noisy machinery may need to be enclosed to reduce noise levels - this may be better for the employee as wearing ear protectors may not be convenient or comfortable. When daily noise levels are at or in excess of 90 dB (A) or peaking above 140 dB (SPL) it is legally mandatory to wear ear protectors and Ear Protection Zones should be clearly marked.

For workers who are regularly exposed to high noise levels there is a duty on the employer to have workers' hearing tested regularly. Records should be kept, the worker informed of the test results and medical advice should be sought if there is hearing loss.

All requirements about noise at work are the responsibility of the UK Government's Health and Safety Executive which has produced a series of useful free leaflets about noise in the workplace. The H&SE contact details are found at the end of this book.

It is common sense to ensure, as much as possible, that ear protectors are kept clean; this will minimise dirt, fungi or bacteria entering the ear canal or adhering to the pinna. Workers in telephone service centres should try, as much as possible, not to use colleagues' headsets and microphones to minimise the risks of cross infection.

In the leisure field there are number of activities, which can especially give rise to participants' hearing loss. These include shooting, playing and listening to music, aircraft and trainspotting, woodworking and modelmaking, grass and tree cutting and driving and racing cars and motorcycles/scooters. With all these activities it is important that the participants think of protecting their hearing. Traditionally, it is highly amplified rock music which has been associated with hearing loss in musicians and the audience; the risk classical musicians who play loud pieces regularly is now being investigated and voluntary limitation of regularly playing loud symphonies is being considered with perspex protective shields being placed within some orchestras.

Parents have a great responsibility in protecting the hearing of their children.They should consider limiting the children's usage of personal music systems and excessive attendance at noisy music, especially heavy rock, concerts. Certainly, parents should not take their new born young babies to a rock concert. This occurrence was reported recently in the newspapers; luckily, the stewards' attention was drawn to the situation and the parents were rightly asked to leave!

It is possible that people who are predisposed to produce a large volume of ear wax when they exercise could consider reducing the amount of exercise that they take. These individuals should weigh up the many advantages of exercise against the disadvantage of possibly producing an excessive amount of wax.

The middle ear

The two main reasons for conductive deafness in the middle ear are the presence of infection, which prevents the eardrum or ossicles bones vibrating correctly, or damage to the ossicle bones themselves.

Infection can be caused by dysfunction/ malfunction of the Eustachian tube. The tube can be helped in its work by swallowing - this can be done whether eating or not. To minimise viral or bacterial infection entering the tube from the upper respiratory tract a healthy lifestyle should be adopted, consisting of elements such as adopting a balanced diet with supplements where necessary, drinking plenty of water, taking regular appropriate exercise, getting plenty of good rest, and reducing the intake of substances like alcohol, tobacco, caffeine and illegal drugs.

Damage to the ossicle bones through arthritis and osteoporosis is difficult to prevent. Factors such as having a sufficient intake of dairy foods, taking an appropriate amount of weight bearing exercise and hormone replacement therapy treatment (especially for vulnerable middle aged women), have to be taken into account.

SENSORINEURAL HEARING LOSS

This type of hearing loss occurs mainly in the cochlear part of the inner ear/ labyrinth, the auditory nerve and the brain.

The cochlea

One of the reasons babies can be born deaf are if diseases such as mumps or rubella (German measles) are contracted by the mother in pregnancy or by a child who has not been inoculated with a preventative vaccine. The question of having a combined MMR (mumps, measles and rubella) inoculation is currently very much in the public domain because of the question of possible adverse side-effects to some children having the combined innoculation.

Exposure to loud noise, either in the short-term or over a long period of time, which can irreversibly damage the cochlea hair cells should be minimised.

The risks of serious head injuries such as skull fractures, which can lead to hearing loss, should be minimised. There is a strict safety code of practice on construction sites, which demands that workers and visitors wear 'hard hats'. In the leisure field, protective headwear is worn by motorcyclists, racing drivers and mechanics trackside; boxers and martial arts fighters; jockeys and other horse riders; climbers and potholers; slalom canoeists and cricket/ baseball batters amongst others. It is vital that officials and those others responsible for supervising potentially dangerous sports activities should check that participants follow the necessary guidelines and rulings.

Hearing loss and blood microcirculation within the ear has been linked to nutrition. Studies at the University of Georgia (1998) linked hearing loss in elderley people with deficiencies in vitamin B12 and folic acid and consequent build up of cholesterol. Other studies have idicated the link between hearing loss and deficiencies in vitamins A, B12 and D, Folic Acid, Iodine, iron, magnesium and zinc.
Strome et al (1988) found that a drop in cholesterol level improved hearing.

The acoustic nerve

The two conditions, which affect the acoustic nerve, are neuromas (benign tumours) and neurofibromatosis (an uncommon inherited disorder characterized by many soft swellings that grow from the nerve). Neither of these conditions is preventable.

The brain

The brain can be affected by a number of conditions. Impaired blood and oxygen supply can be affected by diet, intake of alcohol and smoking. Injury to the brain may be preventable by wearing protective headwear or by wearing seat belts in cars and fast powerboats. Other problems such as infection within the brain, tumours and degeneration are generally not preventable.

Tinnitus

As we have seen in the previous chapter there are two categories of tinnitus; objective and subjective.

Objective tinnitus is a result of a physical malfunction, either in the jaw joint, muscles of the roof of the mouth or blood flow - these causes can be heard by a doctor and are treatable. They are not preventable by an individual.

Subjective tinnitus is a condition, which is difficult to prevent because it can come on without any warning or without any perceptible cause. Of all the causes of tinnitus, which were outlined in the previous chapter, the following are probably the only preventable causes of the condition;

- [ ] head injuries - by wearing protective headwear and following safe work practice
- [ ] catarrh - this could be reduced by following a healthy lifestyle especially reducing on dairy products
- [ ] loud noise - reduce exposure to loud music (live or recorded), wear ear defenders in a noisy workplace, for example in a forge or at a leisure venue, such as a rifle shooting range
- [ ] trigger items - reduce intake of nicotine, caffeine, alcohol and restricted drugs
- [ ] stress - take action to reduce stress at home in the work place, such as by working flexible hours, having longer holidays, receiving counselling or therapies e.g. seated massage, reflexology or yoga
- [ ] ear irrigation/ cleansing (formerly known as syringing) - to avoid the possibility of earwax build up around the eardrum with subsequent cleansing appropriate ear drops, such as sodium bicarbonate or warm olive oil, can be applied to the ear canal
- [ ] introduce zinc supplements - a study by Gersdorff M et al in Belgium found that this gave a significant improvement in continuous tinnitus.

BALANCE PROBLEMS

There are three parts of the body which work together with the brain to affect balance and motion - the eyes; sensory receptors in the skin, muscles and joints; and the vestibule and three semicircular canals (the vestibular sysytem) in the inner ear. Whilst some conditions such as labyrinthitis and Ménière's disease, which both affect balance are not preventable, actions can be taken by individuals to prevent the possibility of dizziness and vertigo arising.

Dizziness
There are a number of causes of dizziness, and some of these causes can be addressed, including;

- [ ] **tiredness** - work and/ or sleep patterns could be changed
- [ ] **stress** - stress relief measures can be put into place
- [ ] **anaemia** - if it is the iron deficiency type of anaemia, foods containing iron such as fruit, wholemeal bread, beans, lean meat and green vegetables can be added to the diet. If it is the megaloblastic type, as well as taking iron rich food, folic acid tablets especially important for pregnant women can also be taken
- [ ] **hypoglycaemia** - this is a low glucose (sugar) level in the blood, a condition that is especially relevant to diabetics. To prevent this condition occurring it is important for the diabetes to be controlled appropriately by the individual. If he/ she is dependent on insulin, sugar should be carried in the form of sugar lumps, chocolate bars or glucose tablets, which can be taken at the first sign of an attack
- [ ] **eye strain** - incorrect working and living conditions such as poor lighting levels may cause eye strain, and it is recommended, if necessary, that the correct glasses or contact lenses are worn with regular eye tests being carried out. Obviously glasses should be kept clean and contact lenses changed when needed.

Vertigo

Vertigo is more serious than dizziness, and is caused by disturbance to either the vestibular part of the inner ear or the vestibular nerve, which goes to the brain. Most of the conditions, which cause vertigo, are not preventable e.g. Ménière's disease, tumours of the brain stem, Multiple Sclerosis and acoustic neuromas.

There are however some causes of vertigo which can be preventable to some extent, these include;

- [ ] avoiding balance disturbing rides at amusement parks or sailing
- [ ] reducing the risk or cervical osteoarthritis - by taking oils such as cod liver oil, as well as adding fish rich in oil, e.g. mackerel or herring, to the diet
- [ ] averting migraine attacks - by isolating triggers to the condition such as specific foods e.g. chocolate or caffeine or stress (or lack of it)
- [ ] overcoming any psychological origin, such as agoraphobia by undertaking hypnosis or other therapies.

Ménière's Disease

This is another inner ear problem which is not preventable. However, once it has been diagnosed a sufferer has a number of different options to reduce its effects which will make his/ her life more bearable and also improve the life of those in close contact - family, friends or colleagues. There are many different steps which could be taken including;

☐   reducing salt in the diet
☐   becoming less stressed
☐   reducing dairy intake
☐   taking Ginkgo Biloba which is a natural herbal product if there is no risk of side effects
☐   having complementary therapies such as acupuncture and ear candles.

Congenital defects

Unless a mother during pregnancy has ignored risks to the baby's health by smoking, drinking alcohol or taking illegal drugs there is nothing preventable in congenital defects. A baby can be born with conditions such as a genetic hereditary nerve deafness or the absence of the pinna, ossicle bones or external ear canal.

Injury to the ear

To avoid repeated injuries to the pinna, contact sports such as boxing or rugby should be given up for something potentially less risky to the ear. Protective headgear should be worn and in rugby this is called a 'scrum cap'.

Tumours

Skin cancers, which affect the ear and areas around the ear, can often be avoided if sufficient protection is taken against excessive exposure to the hot sun's rays. Cancers are most common in pale skinned and fair haired people. The highest incidences of people affected by skin cancer are found in Queensland, Australia and in the Northeast part of Iran. In Australia, the risk of skin cancer is taken so seriously that sunbathers on beaches are warned about the strength of the sun and free sun protection cream is given out. Babies and young children, especially, should wear clothing and hats to protect them from the sun. Care should also be exercised not to use tanning sun beds excessively.

Other skin conditions

As well as cancer, the pinna and the outer ear canal can be affected by a number of other skin conditions. Of these the most common are psoriasis, dermatitis and eczema.

Psoriasis can be improved if stress levels are reduced, the skin is not damaged perhaps by not scratching with an implement and overall illness levels are improved.

Dermatitis is caused by an allergy and can be prevented to some extent, if it is found what is the cause of the problem and the culprit is avoided.

Eczema is also caused by an allergy and can be reduced by finding out what is the allergy and coping with it.

Cholesteatoma

As this is a condition caused by problems with the healing of the ear drum after perforation, the only prevention is to try to ensure that the ear drum doesn't perforate in the first place. The reduction of infection in the tympanic cavity and/or the amount of wax around the ear drum in the external ear canal and reducing exposure to extremely loud noise are ways to possibly prevent perforation.

Poisoning and drugs

While most drugs which can affect the ears are prescribed by doctors there are a couple of common drugs - quinine and aspirin, which are potentially harmful (otoxic) to the ears, which can be purchased and used without doctors' knowledge. It is only likely that if these two drugs are taken in excessive doses that the ear will be damaged by otoxicity. Obviously, these two drugs when taken in a medically recommended dosage will have great benefits for a large number of complaints.

Degeneration

While people can suffer with hearing problems due to the ageing process the best preventative is to follow good guidelines concerning elements such as reducing exposure to loud noise, wearing ear protection and hearing aids when needed.

CHAPTER 7:
CONVENTIONAL TREATMENT OF EAR PROBLEMS

Introduction

As we have already seen there are a large number of problems which affect the ear. These can be loosely defined as hearing problems, balance problems, a combination of balance and hearing problems and other generalized problems.

In this chapter we will look at conventional medical methods of treatment and some self help actions which can be undertaken. In chapter 9 we will examine many of the complementary/alternative therapies which are now available whose aims are to help ear and inner head problems as well as other related conditions.

HEARING PROBLEMS

The outer ear

While medical attention should be sought to remove excessive wax or objects lodged in the outer ear canal it is possible to try to remove an insect by tilting the affected ear so that it is facing upwards. Lukewarm water can then be poured into the ear, and the insect which may be attracted to the light may float to the surface. If this doesn't work, you can consult a General Practitioner doctor at his surgery or visit the hospital casualty (A & E) department. Chloroform, metholated spirits or oil can be used by the doctor to kill an insect if it is alive in the ear, irrigation cleansing will be carried out afterwards.

Ear Irrigation

The main cause of a blockage in the outer ear canal is through wax which has been pushed down towards the ear drum and which in severe cases becomes stuck [impacted] on the drum itself. The description for cleansing the ear canal, which usually takes place in a GP practice, is 'ear irrigation' (previously known as ear syringing). The procedure is normally carried out by a Practice Nurse.

The traditional metal ear syringe should not be used because its design when coupled with the pressure of water it creates within the ear canal renders it inherently dangerous. There is also the problem of correctly sterilising the syringe after every application. Some syringes broke and caused injury during use and the pressure of water applied directly on to the ear drum (tympanic membrane) was often too great.

The introduction of electronic ear irrigators in the United Kingdom in the 1990s, mainly as a response to the number of injuries and consequent litigation, allowed irrigation of the ear canal rather than wax removal under pressure. The medical devices agency (MDA) in London issued Safety Notice SN 9807 in February 1998 which recommended that practitioners use an electronic ear irrigator rather than the manual syringe and refer to the procedure as 'ear irrigation'.

The different irrigators have a variable pressure control which allows the flow of water to be easily controlled with irrigation starting at the minimum setting.

The Propulse II irrigator has specific disinfecting guidelines issued.

The manufacturers of the Multimed - Otoscillo irrigating jet machine don't recommend a specific solution to disinfect the machine (which may lead to inappropriate solutions being used and the machine harbouring infection) and its design doesn't allow the water to be directed to the preferred posterior ear canal wall.

A third possibility - the Welch Allyn Ear Wash System, which is American, attaches to a combined hot and cold water tap. It has the drawback in the United Kingdom that a number of taps in the community, GP and hospital settings are not suitable. While the system cannot be used in rooms without a suitable tap, it does limit the maximum amount of water pressure exerted and controls variation in the flow of water. There is an automatic cut out when there is an increase or decrease in the water temperature. The machine also has a suction system which returns the discharge and debris away from the ear and it can be used without the flow of water to remove any remaining moisture from the ear canal itself.

An excellent document about ear care has been compiled, on behalf of the Action on ENT Steering Board, by Hilary Harkin who is a very experienced nurse based in London. It provides the practitioner (a trained doctor, nurse or audiologist) guidance in otoscopy, ear irrigation, aural toilet, manual wax removal and microsuction. This guidance document in ear care has been endorsed by the Royal College of General Practitioners, Royal College of Nursing, Primary Ear Care Centre Yorkshire and the Medical Devices Agency. As a point of interest, Hilary gained her ear candles therapy qualification with the author in London in 2002.

It is important that before any cleansing procedure is carried out that the consent of the patient is given after the procedure has been fully explained by the practitioner and it is clear that the patient has understood fully what he/she is being told. It may be helpful for the patient to take along a friend or other person as reassurance. This could be especially useful for both the patient and practitioner if the patient has impaired hearing, is nervous or does not have English as a first language.

Electronic irrigation

This is designed to allow the removal of wax and foreign bodies which are not hydroscopic from the ear canal. Hydroscopic matter such as peas and lentils absorb water and expand making removal more difficult. Removal of discharge, keratin and other debris is helped by irrigation.
Irrigation is needed to;
- treat otitis externa when the canal walls are obscured with debris
- improve conduction of sound to the ear drum when it is blocked by wax
- remove debris to allow examination of the ear canal and the ear drum.

Contraindications

There are a number of reasons why the procedure should not be carried out;
● the patient has previously experienced complications in the past after this procedure
● there is a history of middle ear infection in the previous six weeks
● the patient has undergone any form of ear surgery, apart from grommets that have come out at least 18 months previously
● the patient has a perforation or there is a history of mucous discharge in the last year
● patient has a cleft palate (repaired or not)
● in the presence of acute otitis externa with pain and tenderness of the pinna.

Procedure

There are number of steps which should be carried out with this procedure and these include;

● both participants should be seated, the practitioner should use a headlight and head mirror with light source throughout the procedure. The pinna, ear canal and adjacent scalp should be inspected by direct light
● check whether the patient has had ears irrigated previously, if there are any contraindications and explain the procedure to the patient
● the patient should sit in an examination chair with the head tilted toward the affected ear. The patient's shoulder be covered and a bowl placed under the ear to be treated. Check that the temperature of the water is approximately 40°C and set the water pressure to minimum in the machine
● direct water from the tip of the nozzle towards the rear canal wall, the practitioner can periodically inspect the canal with the auriscope/otoscope and inspect the solution running into the bowl
● after removal of the wax or debris, dry mop excess water from the canal using a Jobson Horne probe covered with best quality cotton wool. Examine the ear and give the patient appropriate advice, refer to a doctor if necessary
● always use a clean speculum, jet tip applicator and probe for each patient.

Follow manufacturer guidelines for cleaning and disinfecting all items used during the procedure
● **the procedure should never cause pain, if the patient complains of pain -stop immediately.**

Aural toilet

An aural toilet is used to clear the ear canal of debris, discharge, soft wax or excess fluid following irrigation. The procedure should only be carried out by a trained doctor, nurse or audiologist and an individual assessment should be made of each patient to ensure that he/she is appropriate for aural toilet to be carried out.

Procedure

The ear should be examined and using a Jobson Horne probe and a piece of fluffed up cotton wool, the size of a postage stamp, applied to the probe dry mop the ear. Under direct vision with headlight, or head mirror and light, the pinna should be pulled to straighten the ear canal and the ear cleaned with a gentle rotational action of the probe. The tympanic membrane is not touched.
The cotton wool should be replaced as soon as it becomes soiled. The canal should be re-examined intermittently using the otoscope to check for any remaining items.
Patients who have mastoid cavities should usually be followed up in an ENT department. If the cavity gets repeatedly infected, the patient should be considered for revision surgery.
If any infection is present in the canal, treatment should follow accepted directives and guidelines; if a patient has repeated problems with the ear an ENT surgeon should review them.
Advice should be given to the patient regarding ear care and any relevant information.

The types of wax to be removed

The ear(s) should be examined to ascertain the type of wax to be removed. Is it healthy wax or is it bacterial debris of waxy appearance? Is it dry crumbly wax which could be related to Seborrhoeic Dermatitis? Is it soft, beige wax in both ears which can be associated with high cholesterol?
Hard, crusty wax can often be gently manoeuvred out of the canal with a ring probe with the practitioner using a head mirror or light for illumination. Alternatively a wax hook or forceps can be used. If the treatment becomes painful it should not be continued as the canal lining quickly becomes traumatized with the risk of infection. Cerumenolytic ear drops such as olive oil or sodium bicarbonate should be correctly applied daily for up to one week. Instructions are usually on their container, which often has an applicator dropper. Insertion of the drops could be carried out before going to bed with cotton wool being used as a 'plug' to stop the drops running out of the ear. After one week the patient can return for irrigation or further instrumentation.
Care has to be taken when using any ear drops to break up ear wax because patients may develop irritation from the astringent qualities of some of the agents. This is especially applicable to older adults or people who suffer dermatology conditions or a recurrent otitis externa. If a perforation is suspected behind the ear wax a patient should be advised to use olive oil in very small amounts. **Again any experience of pain should lead to the cessation of use of drops.**
Advice and any other relevant information should be given to the patient regarding ear care.

Microsuction

The use of a microscope and suction is carried out to;
● remove wax and hygroscopic foreign bodies in ears which are not appropriate for irrigation
● remove discharge, keratin or debris from the ear canal or mastoid cavity.

The procedure should be explained beforehand to the patient and they can ask for a rest if they should experience vertigo, if this should occur the patient can focus the eyes on a fixed object until the feeling subsides. The suction generates loud noise and sometimes heat and the patient should be advised beforehand that this will happen.

The magnification, eye piece and angle of the microscope can be adjusted. The patient should position him/herself comfortably on the examination couch or chair.
The pinna, canal and adjacent scalp are examined by direct light to check for incision scars or skin defects.

The pinna is moved so that the ear canal can be straightened. A speculum is placed gently into the canal and the suction tip with suction tubing attached is thread down the canal. The suction tip is used, at a pressure of 80-120mm Hg/18-20 cm H2O to remove the debris and if the tubing becomes blocked it can be washed through. The intention is only to touch the debris not the walls of the canal cavity or ear drum. The practitioner regularly inspects all parts of the canal, cavity, ear drum or drum remnant by using the microscope. The condition of the ear canal is checked when removing the speculum and appropriate advice should be given to the patient about ear care and other related matters.

The Presence of Infection in the outer ear canal

If there is infection in this part of the ear it can be treated in different ways depending on its nature. If it is localised, it can be treated with analgesics or oral antibiotics. **No aspirin should be prescribed to those less than 16 years of age.** If the infection is acute and diffused and not fungal then a preparation like 'Earcalm' can be used. If the condition does not respond to treatment a swab should be taken and referral made to a specialist practitioner.

Damage to the ear drum

Most ear drum perforations, except when a grommet is surgically inserted, are due to acute infection or injury and heal quite quickly, usually within a month. If the perforation fails to heal or close completely within six months a myringoplasty/tympanoplasty (ear drum repair) operation is carried out. Tissue is sewn on to the surface of the ear drum and the graft is usually taken from the fibrous covering of a muscle in the temple or the thigh.

The middle ear

There are two reasons for conductive hearing loss in the middle ear;
- **otosclerosis** affecting the stapes (stirrup) ossicle bone which prevents it vibrating correctly
- **the presence of infection**, especially glue ear, which can stop all the three ossicle bones vibrating.

Otosclerosis

This is a disorder that often causes progressive deafness. It can be hereditary and about one person in 200 can be affected. It usually starts in early adulthood and hearing loss progresses for 10- 15 years. It is more common in women than men and it often develops during pregnancy. Sound is muffled and is more pronounced when there is background noise. It is diagnosed when there are abnormal results in hearing tests. Whilst hearing aids can significantly improve the condition it can only be cured by a stapedectomy - an operation when the stapes/stirrup bone, which has become overgrown and fused to the incus/anvil bone is replaced by an artificial substitute which will take over its role as acting as a piston at the labyrinth's oval window.

If both ears are affected usually only one ear will be treated at a time because of possible risks. All or most of the bone is removed and it is replaced by a plastic or metal prosthesis which resembles a shepherd's crook. One end is inserted into the entrance to the inner ear, and the other end is hooked on to the incus (middle ossicle) bone. This operation, which can be carried out under local anaesthetic takes about one hour at an approximate cost of £2,500 (February 2004 price) and improves hearing considerably in 90% of cases. Aftercare can be a night in hospital and the prescription of paracetemol. However, there can be side effects to this operation, as in all surgical cases, and there is a possibility of facial weakness if it is carried out under local anaesthetic.

When you consider the minute size of these bones and other parts of the total ear, nose and throat environment you realise how skilled specialist practitioners and surgeons are in their work and the length of time and dedication it must take to train to high standards.

Sometimes hearing aids can be used to lessen deafness which can be caused by otosclerosis. The hearing aid may take the form of a device which transmits sound to the inner ear through a vibrating pad which touches the bone behind the ear.

The presence of infection
Glue ear

Although the vast majority of cases of glue ear correct themselves without medical intervention; conventional treatments if necessary are either drugs or surgery. The benefits of antibiotics are only short-term, and antihistamines and decongestants have no proven benefit although they are prescribed in mild cases.

The most common surgical operation (a myringotomy) is to make a hole in the ear drum into which a grommet (most commonly, a small hollow Teflon plastic drainage tube) is placed. This normally takes only a few minutes to perform under local or general anaesthetic as a day case or on an in-patient basis depending on individual circumstances. Not only will it allow infected fluid to drain out into the outer ear canal, but it will also allow air into the middle ear, hence avoiding a further build-up of fluid. There are different types of grommet for different purposes. Most grommets stay in place for 6-12 months before falling out but some are meant to stay in the ear drum for a longer period. They are designed to fall outwards into the ear canal but very rarely they have been known to fall backwards into the tympanic cavity behind the ear drum.

Often a specialist may recommend removing the adenoids at the same time as inserting the grommet as this can help prevent the recurrence of glue ear and it may help prevent colds and other infections. Removal of adenoids necessitates an overnight stay in hospital.

A modern alternative form of surgery is laser myringotomy because it can be done without a general anaesthetic which has its advantages for those who cannot tolerate a general anaesthetic. Currently, many adults have a grommet fitted after having a local anaesthetic cream applied to the ear.

Sometimes, grommets have to be reinserted because the condition reappears. With insertion or reinsertion there is a risk of scarring to the ear drum, which may have consequences later in life, for instance when ear irrigation takes place, or infection if water gets near the grommet. Patients should wear earplugs when showering or bathing and swimmers should also wear a tight fitting cap.

For about half of all children who have glue ear the condition clears up on its own, within this period it is important to deal sympathetically with the child. Before having an operation a child could try to clear the Eustachian tube by blowing up a special balloon from the nostrils - older children are usually better at this technique.

Other middle ear infections

Acute otitis media can be treated with antibiotic drugs and painkillers (analgesics).

Inflammation can result from a viral or bacterial upper respiratory tract infection extending up the Eustachian tube into the post tympanic cavity, antibiotics can be prescribed.

Inflammation might also be caused by enlarged adenoids. To check for enlarged adenoids, a doctor usually inspects the back of the throat using a mirror with a light attached; sometimes an x-ray may be taken. Infections usually respond to antibiotics, but if they recur frequently an adenoidectomy (the surgical removal of the adenoids) may be recommended. In most cases the inflammation will clear itself, however complications can include inflammation of the outer ear, damage to the ossicle bones exacerbating deafness, or a cholesteatoma. The cholesteatoma can be life threatening and can cause mastoiditis or a brain tumour and has to be surgically removed.

The inner ear

It is in this part of the ear that sensorineural deafness occurs. This form of deafness cannot be cured because structures are extremely delicate and surgery cannot be performed on them. However, hearing aids can be used to increase the volume of sound reaching the inner ear by means of an amplifier and an earphone which fits in the outer ear canal. The subject of hearing aids is covered in depth in chapter 10.

Cochlear implants

Another technical aid for the treatment of sensorineural deafness is a cochlear implant, in which electrodes that can receive sound signals are surgically implanted in the inner ear. This advance which is an extremely expensive procedure needing a large amount of on- going treatment by therapists in different disciplines has been greeted with mixed reactions. The implants have been particularly successful in helping children born profoundly deaf to learn how to speak and hear.

A cochlear implant is a relatively new type of electronic device which is implanted within the cochlea part of the labyrinth/inner ear to help people with very severe or total sensorineural hearing loss caused by damage to the cochlea hair cells. Their cochlear nerve is intact. Some users hear very well and can use a telephone normally, others may not be as successful, but they can hear environmental sounds like dogs barking or birds singing. Most people find that implant assisted hearing improves their lip reading and conversation becomes easier even if they cannot understand speech through hearing alone.

How does a cochlear implant work?

A small part of the device is surgically implanted in the cochlea to electrically stimulate the cochlear/acoustic nerve - this gives the sensation of hearing. Another part, the speech processor which is externally worn, is connected to a headpiece with a microphone to pick up the sound waves. The processor converts the sound waves into electrical signals. The headpiece has a transmitter which sends the signals through the skin to the receiver and then to the implant. The transmitter is held in place over the internally implanted receiver (above the pinna) by a magnet.

A wire leads down from the receiver through the middle ear and then into the cochlea. An implant can have up to twenty two electrodes and these are located along the part of the wire called the electrode array, this is then threaded into the cochlea.

The electrical signals are sent from the processor to the electrodes. The electrodes simulate the action of the hair cells, so the electrodes at the beginning of the electronic array are stimulated by high frequencies and those at the end of the array (near the apex of the cochlea) are stimulated by low frequencies. The signals are then passed along the cochlear nerve to the brain's auditory centre where they are decoded as hearing. Advances in design have led to an implant which can stimulate the cochlear nerve 83,000 times each second and it will be possible to increase this stimulation process in the future.

Who is suitable for a cochlear implant?
Cochlear implants are suitable for adults and children who have severe to profound sensorineural deafness in both ears and cannot get significant benefit from conventional hearing aids. There are different constraints for adults, teenagers and children;

- **adults** - there is no upper age barrier to having an implant fitted and while they are suitable for those who have been deaf for years and those who have become deafened recently they may benefit more adults born partially deaf who then had a progressive loss because they have memory of sound
- **teenagers** - can benefit most if deafness occurs after acquiring speech and language or who have been born with impaired hearing and are good hearing aid users. A cochlear implant may be better than a hearing aid for a severely deaf person
- **children** - about 840 children are born with a significant hearing loss in the UK each year (source: Defeating Deafness charity); 400 of these will be profoundly or severely deaf and about 200 will receive implants (from a report 'Cochlear Implants' published by the National Cochlear Implant Users Association, UK). Whilst implants will not cure deafness they should allow children who have one to perform better and their results are more like those of a severely deaf child rather than of a profoundly deaf child. The decision to fit an implant to suitable deaf children is opposed by some deaf parents who want their children to be part of the deaf community and learn to sign. This controversial question has to be addressed on an individual basis. If children are implanted, best results are achieved from a young age - one to three years old. Parents of children deafened by meningitis should seek expert advice urgently as it may be difficult to insert the implant if the cochlea becomes filled with tiny (ossified) bone which may be the result of this condition. There is a follow up programme for children and a team of experts including an educational psychologist and local teachers of the Deaf.

What are the criteria for an implant?
The following criteria apply to adults and teenagers being considered for an implant;
- Have satisfactory physical and mental health
- Have good support from family and friends
- Get little or no benefit from conventional hearing aids with well fitting moulds
- Be able to attend the cochlear implant centre for tuning and follow up sessions.

Before deciding to have an implant fitted it may be useful to meet an implant user or the family of a child user to talk about its benefits or any problems which may have occurred.

What are the benefits of an implant?
Like all other treatments the benefit of an implant varies from person to person. Factors which affect the success of the procedure include;
- damage to the auditory nerve
- whether the cochlea has ossified with bony fragments preventing the insertion of all the electrodes into the cochlea
- the length of time someone has been deaf.

Positive results of having an implant fitted include;
- the world becomes less dangerous because a Deaf person can hear sirens and other warning signals. The implant will not tell someone from which direction a noise is coming as it takes both ears to do this
- helping lip -reading and possibly obviating the need to lip read
- the voice can be used more confidently with variance of tone and volume
- probable improvement of tinnitus because the sound from the implant masks the tinnitus
- possible enjoyment of music by wearers.

Assessment and testing of someone who wants an implant

Someone who thinks a cochlea implant would be beneficial has to take the following route;
1. contact the doctor (GP)
2. referral to a local hospital ENT consultant
3. referral to a cochlear implant centre
4. see a team of other professionals including implant centre consultant, audiological scientist, speech and language therapist, hearing therapist, and possibly a clinical psychologist or counsellor and a social worker with Deaf people. If there is a problem in being referred, the implant centre can be approached directly.

The following tests may be carried out when assessing someone for an implant;
- audiological tests to measure hearing and determine the most suitable ear for the implant
- CT or MRI scans of the inner ear
- electrical tests to check the condition of the acoustic nerve
- psychological tests
- a trial with the most powerful hearing aid to determine the benefit of conventional amplification.

As soon as a decision to go ahead is taken there may be a wait of up to 18 months depending on which health authority is going to fund the operation and the length of the waiting list of other people wanting the operation. We have seen that the implant will cost £18,500 and rehabilitation will cost a further £15,000.

The operation to fit a cochlear implant and the follow up sessions

The operation, which is performed under general anaesthetic, requires a hospital stay of two or three days, with the patient returning after a week for a check up. The implant is turned on and tuned by the audiologist after six weeks to allow the post operative swelling to go down. In the first year there are several follow up visits with further tuning and a rehabilitation programme is put into place. After this only annual visits are needed unless there are any problems or the equipment needs emergency repairs.

In the USA it is recommended that inoculation against bacterial meningitis is considered prior to the operation as the introduction of a foreign body (the implant) may lead to a risk of this condition. The UK Government in 2002 followed the same line when it recommended that all cochlear implant users have vaccination against pneumococcal meningitis.

It is important that a user perseveres with the implant and that it is worn as much as possible. Sometimes benefits will come quickly; sometimes it takes months for an improvement. If an internal part fails it can be replaced. If a wearer decides to have the implant removed this can be done.

It is important that those supporting someone in the family fitted with an implant realise that much of the success of the procedure will be due to helping the individual by actions such as reading out loud and helping with homework. Information and advice about cochlear implants can be given by the National Cochlear Implant Users Association (contact details at the end of this book).

The acoustic nerve

With an acoustic nerve neuroma, which is a benign tumour of nerve tissue, the traditional treatment has been radiotherapy which can be costly, and emotionally damaging to the patient. An advanced technique which has been used to good effect in Sheffield, England is a technique known as the 'Sheffield Gamma Knife'. In this procedure 201 gamma rays with cobalt sources are directed at lesions in the brain. Different types of tumours including neuromas are treated. Worldwide, 100,000 patients have been treated since 1985 using this procedure.

The Gamma - Knife can treat either unilateral or bilateral tumours up to 3 cms maximum diameter. The aim is to prevent tumour growth, rather than complete removal; hopefully preserving residual hearing which is often followed by substantial shrinkage. While managing progressive neuromas, cranial nerve function is preserved - acoustic, facial and trigeminal nerves. Intensive post-operative care of the patient has to be undertaken including ITU ventilation and careful nursing observation.
If the facial nerve is affected by the procedure (1% in typical small surgery and up to 30% in large surgery) and palsy develops a facial nerve stimulator can be applied.
In Britain, a second similar unit has been established at the Cromwell private hospital, Kensington, West London.

Single sided deafness (SSD)
Another type of surgical intervention being pioneered by Mr David Proops, Consultant ENT Surgeon at the Queen Elizabeth Hospital Birmingham, England for people who unfortunately have single sided deafness (SSD), due to damage to the acoustic nerve after surgery to remove a benign tumour, is to have a bone-anchored hearing aid (BAHA) fitted. In this new type of operation, which is carried out under local anaesthetic and which takes 45 minutes - one hour, a small hole is drilled in the mastoid bone and in this is fitted a seat for a hearing device attachment which is fitted later. Sound is re-routed via direct skull bone conduction to the cochlea in the other ear.

This contrasts to a normal hearing aid which amplifies sound in the same ear. So far the operation has had a 95-97% success rate and the cost is £5,000 - £7,000 (October 2003 price), more details can be obtained from the British Acoustic Neuroma Association. It is estimated that 9,000 people are affected by SSD in the UK each year.

Tinnitus

As we have already seen tinnitus is an extremely complex problem which is brought about by a number of, or a single trigger factor. So far there have been no cures for tinnitus but there are a number of steps which can be followed to reduce its impact on an individual who is a sufferer.

The initial step is to contact his/her doctor. The doctor will check the ears and possibly determine that tinnitus is a symptom of another condition that may be treatable with drugs, for example if there is an outer or middle ear infection antibiotics may be prescribed to clear the infection which may in turn improve the tinnitus. A decongestant or antihistamine, prescribed by the doctor may also help to clear a blocked nose which may again help the tinnitus. A GP or practice nurse may clear the outer ear canal of impacted wax as this may be aggravating the situation.

The GP may also feel that a certain drug such as aspirin or a specific antibiotic may be contributing to the tinnitus. Advice should always be sought from a doctor before any medication is changed, dosage altered or given up.

Often the doctor will refer patients to the local hospital ENT department which may have its own tinnitus clinic or know of one locally. The specialist in an ENT department or clinic may suggest a number of different treatment options;

- **hearing aids** which may pick up sounds we don't know we hear which will distract the brain from the tinnitus. It may also help the brain to stop straining to hear and it is this straining which can make the brain focus on the tinnitus noises
- **sound therapy** is also known as sound enrichment/enhancement. Often the tinnitus is more noticeable in a quiet environment. The therapy works by filling silent times with pleasant noise - sea sounds, television, music or a sound generator (formerly known as a noise masker). Often sounds and music are available on cassette, CD or CD Rom. The therapy can help sleeping. A wearable noise generator (WNG) resembles, and can be combined with, a hearing aid and gives a 'shushing'noise which deflects attention away from the tinnitus. It is a constant, wide-band noise at a level (around 2000Hz) just quieter than the tinnitus. It is worn as much as possible, either in or behind the ear, especially during quieter periods for between 6 and 36 months. Generators can also be placed under a pillow or at the bedside for use at night and to supplement one which is worn during the day. Generators are sometimes available on the NHS and can be bought privately.
- **counselling** can help with the understanding and management of the condition
- **relaxation techniques** can help a sufferer relax. Methods can include meditation, Reiki, Yoga, sport, hobbies, social activities and better time management

A new device designed to help tinnitus sufferers is the 'Aurex 3 plus Tinnitus Therapy Device' which is manufactured by Shrewsbury Medical Limited, UK. This machine uses sound synthesis techniques with digital display of its characteristics which enables the sufferer to generate a sound source closely matching the 'perceived' tinnitus sound. The sound source is then externally applied by an electromechanical transducer to the auditory system such that it directly excites the cochlea. This has been shown to reduce/alleviate the symptoms of tinnitus, or in some cases effect a cure.

Habituation (retraining) therapy: Tinnitus Retraining therapy (TRT)

Habituation therapy reduces a reaction to tinnitus so that it becomes less of a problem. Often in the early stages sufferers cannot cope with their new found problem and the effects can seem so bad that suicides can happen. The treatment options shown previously should help speed up the natural process. Other aids can be;
● use complementary therapies such as massage, reflexology, ear candles or acupuncture to balance the body and help relaxation and sleep
● try to listen to a low level of background noise e.g. bird noise, a fan or music (possibly tuned off station)
● do not try to use loud noise to cover the tinnitus as this can exacerbate the problem
● obtain advice from a specialist organisation such as the RNID Tinnitus Helpline, British Tinnitus Association or a local tinnitus support group.

Reducing the effects of tinnitus

Although the effects of tinnitus fluctuate they normally improve over time. Sufferers could consider the following self help actions;
● reduce the time spent listening to loud music - live or recorded
● wear appropriate ear protection in a noisy workplace or at leisure but do not use protectors to shut out everyday sounds
● reduce caffeine and alcohol intake as these may be triggers
● take Gingko Biloba and supplements to improve blood flow to the inner ear, but first check that there will be no effects on any other medication being taken e.g Warfarin or aspirin for blood thinning.

BALANCE PROBLEMS

We have already seen that there are a large number of medical conditions which have dizziness and vertigo as their symptoms. The three main parts of the body which are involved with the brain in the process of balance and movement are the eyes; vestibular part of the inner ear; and sensors in the skin, muscles and joints.

Some of the conditions which lead to imbalance such as a viral infection (labyrinthitis) in the inner ear can be successfully treated with antibiotic drugs; other conditions such as Ménière's Disease can only be controlled using different methods including drugs. Many of the controllable conditions need a large amount of self help, which is covered in chapter 10, which calls for a large amount of discipline.

Dizziness

The treatment of dizziness varies greatly according to its cause. Some causes are relatively easy to treat, others are complicated;

- **postural hypotension** - which is common in the elderly and those on antihypertensive drugs to treat high blood pressure - often occurs when sufferers get up quickly from a lying or sitting position. The treatment is to arise slowly
- **transient ischaemic attacks** (a stroke lasting less than 24 hours) - aim is to reduce a major stroke happening, which may occur within five years, by improving lifestyle with reduction of consumption of alcohol, tobacco and fatty foods. Treatments can be endarterectomy (removal of an artery affected by atherosclerosis - narrowing by deposits of fatty material), anticoagulant drugs or aspirin (which reduces the stickiness of platelets in the blood)
- **tiredness** - the causes of tiredness should be addressed e.g. anxiety, depression, overwork or anaemia
- **stress** - the causes of stress should be addressed, including relaxation techniques and working/leisure activities
- **anaemia** - there are a number of different types of anaemia and preliminary diagnosis of the condition is from the patient's symptoms and the measurement of a low level of haemoglobin. The most common form of anaemia is a lack of iron which is an essential part of haemoglobin. Treatments for the different types of anaemia include bone marrow transplant, removal of the spleen, immunosuppressant drugs, iron injections and tablets (syrup for children), courses of B12 vitamin injections or folic acid (especially important for pregnant women) and iron rich foods such as fruit, liver, wholemeal bread, beans and green vegetables
- **hypoglycaemia** - this occurs when there is an abnormally low level of glucose (sugar) in the blood. People with insulin-dependent diabetes mellitus are those most at risk. The treatment is either for the person to eat sugar lumps, glucose or chocolate. If a person is unconscious a doctor will give an injection of either glucose solution or glucagon hormone
- **eye strain** - if necessary, correct glasses or lenses should be worn and vision should be checked every couple of years in adulthood by an optician or opthalmologist. Correct lighting should be installed in the workplace and in leisure facilities. Sometimes sinusitis, rhinitis, blepharitis (inflammation of the eyelid margins) and conjunctivitis can cause irritation to the eyes and these conditions should be treated with a variety of drugs including antihistamines and eye - drops. The wearing of bifocal spectacles, especially by older people, will often lead to balance problems - if this is the case avoid wearing this type of spectacles
- **subdural haemorrhage** (between the outer two membranes which cover the brain) - surgical drilling into the skull will drain a blood clot and repair damaged blood vessels.

Dizziness is an occasional side effect of most prescribed drugs, especially those which affect circulation including high and low blood pressure.

Vertigo

Vertigo, which is a condition distinct from dizziness, is sometimes caused by conditions which can also cause dizziness. As we saw in chapter 5, there are a large number of bodily conditions which have vertigo as one of its symptoms.
Treatments for some of the causes of conditions which cause vertigo include;

- **Labyrinthitis** - viral causes of an infection of the inner ear usually clear up without treatment but symptoms can be eased by antihistamine drugs such as meclozine. Bacterial causes are treated with antibiotics to prevent infection spreading which may cause permanent deafness or meningitis (inflammation of the meninges (membranes) covering the brain). Surgery may be done to clear any pus or to remove any cholesteatoma
- **Ménière's Disease** - this will be covered in depth later in this chapter
- **cervical (neck area) osteoarthritis** - anti- inflammatory drugs can be prescribed, neck brace can be worn, general heat can be applied and supervised exercise (under the direction of a chartered physiotherapist) can be undertaken. Sufferers can learn to move their necks gently and smoothly
- **tumour of the brain stem** - surgery is an option. Radiotherapy or anticancer drugs can also be given. Corticosteroid drugs are often prescribed to reduce the swelling of tissue around the tumour with a temporary relief of symptoms
- **Multiple Sclerosis** - this can be treated with the drug Interferon which slows the progress of the disease. Corticosteroid drugs can alleviate the symptoms of an acute attack and other drugs can be used to control symptoms such as incontinence and depression. Physiotherapy and other exercises can strengthen muscles and aids and equipment can help maintain mobility
- **Meningitis** (when the acoustic nerve is affected) - this inflammation of the covering of the brain and spinal cord is diagnosed by a lumbar puncture. If its cause is viral this is usually mild and no treatment is necessary; if it is bacterial in origin it is seen as a medical emergency and is treated with intravenous antibiotic drugs
- **Narrowing of the blood vessels which supply oxygen and blood to the brain** - as well as treatment by surgery it is important to adopt a healthy lifestyle to reduce the risk of damage to the brain through a stroke e.g. reduce tobacco and alcohol intake and follow a good diet regime
- **Migraine** - treatment is for the two distinct types of migraine - common and classical which have different symptoms. If migraines occur less than one per month, treatment is for the acute attack; aspirin or paracetemol, plus possibly an antemetic drug can be taken. If these are not successful then sumatripan (which acts on the blood vessels in and around the brain) or ergotamine can be prescribed. Ergotamine can be useful in preventing an attack if taken before a headache begins. If migraine attacks are more frequent, prophylactic (disease preventing) drugs are prescribed; beta- blocker drugs or calcium channel blockers. Usually an effective treatment programme can be devised but if the symptoms persist a specialist migraine clinic should be consulted.

Treatment of Benign Paroxysmal Positional Vertigo (BPPV)

Half the cases of BPPV will get better without treatment although the recovery period may be several months. Cases which do not get better within a few weeks can be treated with different particle repositioning manoeuvres such as the Epley manoeuvre. This takes about eight minutes and is designed to reposition free floating chalk particles especially in the posterior or anterior semi-circular canals back into the vestibule. This treatment often brings instant relief to over 90% of patients and two or three additional treatments will help many of the remaining patients.

Some particles may however still be free floating and liable to fall back into the semicircular canals; if this happens a further bout(s) of BPPV may occur at any time. The Epley manoeuvre can be repeated and patients and/or their relatives can be taught how to do it for themselves.

If the chalk crystals become attached to a different part of the jelly in the semicircular canal the bouts of vertigo will last longer (up to two minutes) and the condition will have to be treated with different positioning manoeuvres and exercises.

Anyone who thinks that they suffer with BPPV should ask their GP to refer them to the local hospital ENT/Audiology Department for treatment. As BPPV is a mechanical disorder drugs have no effect except that they may combat the nausea accompanying the worst cases.

Certain antibiotic drugs which are used to treat serious or life- threatening infections can damage the balance organs; it is important to balance the risks of taking/not taking medication.

Exercise treatment

Balance retraining physiotherapy (or similar professional) exercises can help individuals improve their balance if it has been impaired. These could be from a set list such as the Cawthorne-Cooksey exercises, or specific exercises devised for each individual's needs. The patient will be able to do these at his/her own pace without feeling sick or dizzy. It may be several weeks before any improvement is felt - persevere with them!!!
General exercise is also important in helping improve balance; the more enjoyable it is the easier it will be to keep it up.

Cognitive behavioural therapy (CBT)

Someone with a long history of balance problems is likely to be anxious, depressed and suffer from panic attacks. It is important to deal with these emotional issues as well as the causes of the balance problems. If CBT is offered as part of the patient's therapy treatment it allows more control of the symptoms especially when they cause anxiety, CBT is also based on how an individual relates to the environment and treatment can be more specific than traditional forms of behavioural therapy.

Ménière's Disease

Treatment of Ménière's Disease

Because sufferers may not experience all the symptoms of the disease it is important that the treatment regime is specific to each person. Other complications are that there may be periods of remission from the symptoms and they can also be of varied severity at different times. Emotional factors play an important role and a reassuring doctor may help bring about remission periods.

Treatment of the causes of Ménière's Disease can either be dietary, drug orientated or surgery. Amelioration of the effects of its symptoms can often be self help by a sufferer of the condition; these are covered in detail in chapter 10 which covers health self help in general.

Dietary changes

Salt and sodium, which is often used as a preservative, can cause fluid retention and increase endolymphatic pressure (in the inner ear) and their intake should be reduced wherever possible. A reduction in salt may also help with other conditions associated with the kidneys, blood pressure, the heart and brain e.g. strokes. The level of fluid intake should be discussed with a qualified practitioner. Caffeine intake (high in coffee and cola drinks and present in tea) should be reduced to reduce endolymph production.

In the UK diuretics are not used extensively in the management of Ménière's Disease: in the United States this is the opposite case. Diuretics should only be taken under medical supervision. Some are ototoxic (which increases damage to the ears) and others can damage the kidneys. Thiazes are the most commonly used and are the safest but can give disturbance to fluids and electrolytes in the body with a loss of potassium; they can precipitate diabetes. Some patients can benefit from short courses, especially women around the time of their periods.

Drug treatments
Serc (a Betahistine hydrochloride) helps many sufferers by having a direct action on the endolymph production in the inner ear possibly by improving blood flow in small blood vessels. It is important to combine it with a salt free diet for a long period, initially over several months. Dosage can be up to 32mg three times daily. Because it is a histamine preparation which may aggravate symptoms of peptic ulceration it is not prescribed for people with dyspeptic symptoms. Serc can be taken on a long-term basis.

Stemetil (a Prochlorperazine) an anti-vertigo drug which acts as a vestibular sedative is prescribed for patients who have severe attacks of vertigo and dizziness as well as Ménière's Disease. Although it can be given by injection or tablets it can also be applied in suppository form as tablets cannot be absorbed during an attack. It is not usual to take Stemetil on a long-term basis as it damps down a good ear if there is asymmetry. After a while a patient feels better and comes off the drug and the asymmetry returns.

Buccastem is a form of Stemetil which is placed inside the upper lip and absorbed through the mucous membrane. There is a risk of Parkinsonian symptom- like tremor or rigidity developing, especially in older patients as the drug is eliminated slowly from the body and can accumulate over a long period. There are many other anti- vertigo tablets available.

Another prescribed drug is Stugeron (a Cinnarizine) which acts on small blood vessels and prevents constriction on these vessels with an improved micro- circulation in the ear. While it is a mild antihistamine many patients claim benefit from using it (others claim benefit from using histamines!).

Surgery

While sufferers of Ménière's Disease can display a wide range of symptoms there are a number of surgical interventions which can be considered and what works for one person may have no beneficial effects for another;

- A **Saccus Decompression** is an operation which can be performed on the endolymphatic sac which reduces the pressure of the inner ear fluid by extending the bony space surrounding the inner ear, sometimes there is an insertion of a small drainage tube. This is effective in about 80% of patients (Ménière's Society information sheet 1.3.0) especially in the early stages of the disease. Hearing is preserved or improved with little risk
- A **Vestibular Neurectomy** is a major intra-cranial operation which is aimed at abolishing dizziness, involving dividing the vestibular nerve of balance while leaving the acoustic nerve of hearing intact
- A **Labyrinthectomy** is a safe operation which removes the balance part of the inner ear. While it abolishes vertigo it also causes total hearing loss in the affected ear; tinnitus is not affected. Often patients who have this operation or a Vestibular Neurectomy have a post-operative imbalance which can take months to clear
- **Intratympanic injections of Gentamicin** (an aminoglycoside antibiotic) for properly selected patients can be carried out, they do not work for everyone and certainly not for those with bilateral Ménière's
- **A round window catheter operation** can be carried out which should improve spinning and sickness
- **Rehabilitation of hearing** can be achieved by **introducing either a Bone Anchored Hearing Aid** for single sided deafness which conducts sound through bone from the affected to the good side, or **implanting a cochlear implant** in those who have no hearing. This latter group include those who may have had a labyrinthectomy or a vestibular neurectomy. As a comparison a cochlear implant costs £18,500 to buy and £15,000 for patient rehabilitation; a Bone Anchored Hearing Aid costs £2,000 (source: Mr A F O'Connor MB ChB FRCS Consultant Otolaryngologist at Guy's & St Thomas' Hospital, London)

- **A grommet can be inserted in the ear drum**. While the insertion may just be a placebo effect, it is increasingly thought that equalising pressure between the middle and inner ear is important. Changes in the endolymphatic pressure which are associated with typical spinning attacks may be reduced with the insertion of a grommet. The procedure certainly helped the author's partner who suffers with Ménière's Disease, especially the feeling of 'fullness in the ear' she often experiences.

Balance Retraining Exercises (vestibular rehabilitation)

Balance retraining exercises (vestibular rehabilitation) and stress reduction methods which help to control the symptoms of vertigo are useful for some sufferers but are only available at a few specialist centres. The exercises help the brain to cope with movements which induce dizziness. Dizziness and imbalance will be improved between attacks of vertigo and confidence to cope with an attack of vertigo should be enhanced. Booklets about self-help for balance and stress are now available from the Ménière's Society (contact details at the back of the book).

Eye exercises, which are specific to the individual's needs, are designed to improve the vestibular ocular reflex (VOR). They should be linked to other remedial problems such as improving activity levels or helping bad necks or headaches. Both static (standing balance) and dynamic (moving) balance improvements should be goals and when combined they should help improve the quality of life.

At the York District Hospital, UK a successful pilot scheme, based on principles developed in the USA, has been run using an Extended Scope Practitioner (ESP) Chartered Physiotherapist as the key person who looks after patients with dizziness and balance problems. A service is offered which crosses traditional speciality and professional boundaries. The result has been a one-stop clinic run by the physiotherapist and an audiologist. A consultant is also involved in the process but his/her time is saved with financial benefits. There is also a reduction in the number of unnecessary hospital visits and access times are improved. Even with all its advantages, long term funding has still to be secured from the relevant local health care commissioners.

Current research
There is much promising research being carried out throughout the world into Ménière's Disease. This includes including vestibular testing - Head Impulse Testing where the semi-circular canals are tested by short, rapid head movements. Also the newly developed Meniett device has a probe delivering low pressure pulses to the ear of a patient who had a grommet inserted before using the device. It is thought that the pulses reduce excess fluid in the ear with a reduction in dizziness.

Patulous Eustachian Tube (PET)

As we saw in Chapter 5, PET is a condition where the Eustachian tube remains open rather than in its normal closed position (except when it is needed to be open). Like many ear conditions it displays symptoms which can be attributed to other conditions and while diagnosis can be made on history alone it can often be misdiagnosed.

Physical examination and testing of PET

Often examination findings are usual with canals and ear drums appearing normal, except that the ear drum can be atrophic (shrunk or wasted away) due to constant drum motion due to excessive breathing of sniffing. The movement of the ear drum is exaggerated due to forced respiration or with breathing through the nose with one nostril occluded (obstructed). The drum moves medially on inspiration and laterally on expiration. When the patient is sitting up, the pars flaccida (loose) part of the drum moves slightly; this ceases when the patient lies down. These drum movements can be examined with an operating microscope.

Other tests can be carried out to diagnose PET including;
- CT scanning
- Radiology
- Tympanometry
- Microphone testing in the ear canal and linked to the nasal vestibule (sonotubometry)
- Regular monitoring of the middle ear pressure
- Direct nasopharyngoscopy which may show the continuous presence of a triangular opening of the tube.

Treatment of PET

Patients who are pregnant (and their symptoms usually go after delivery) and those with mild symptoms need advice and reassurance only. Patients can be advised to;
- Increase or regain weight
- Avoid diuretics
- Recline or lower the head when symptoms happen
- Apply nasal drops - with anticholingerics or oestrogen.

There are a number of surgical techniques available depending on the cause of PET and they include;
- Insufflation (blowing in) of a solution of salicylic acid and boric acid; repeat treatments are necessary
- Tube diathermy (heat) with probe
- Cauterisation with silver nitrate
- Injection with paraffin, Teflon or Gelfoam
- Transaction of tensor veli palatini muscle
- Myringotomy and insertion of a ventilating tube.

Congenital defects of the ear

Deformities such the absence of, or other structural problem with, the pinna, external ear canal or ossicles have to be dealt with surgically.

Injury to the outer ear

The best form of treatment is prevention rather than cure. Good quality jewellery such as earrings should be used and the hole in the lobe made cleanly. Inflammation of the helix can be treated by steroid injections or in severe cases, surgical excision.

Sportsmen and women should wear protective headgear. If an ear swells after an injury, due to blood collecting between the skin and the underlying cartilage, a cloth wrung out in cold water or an ice pack is used to reduce the swelling. If a doctor thinks it necessary, blood can be drained from the ear (aspirated) using a needle and syringe with a pressure bandage then being applied. If there are repeated injuries with a severely distorted ear, plastic surgery is often necessary.

CHAPTER 8: OTHER INNER HEAD PROBLEMS

Introduction

Having looked at the anatomy, physiology and pathology of the ears in depth we shall in this chapter look at many of the conditions of the nose, throat and surrounding structures together with a view on headaches and migraines as these conditions are often experienced by sufferers of ear, nose and throat problems. Treatment of these problems are covered both in this, and subsequent, chapters.

The conditions to be covered are;
- **Sinusitis**
- **Rhinitis (commonly known as 'Hay fever')**
- **Snoring**
- **Sleep apnoea**
- **Headaches**
- **Migraine**
- **Motion Sickness**
- **Nasal polyps**
- **Facial neuralgia**
- **Bell's palsy**
- **Other conditions causing facial paralysis**
- **Common cold and influenza**
- **Laryngitis**
- **Tonsillitis**
- **Adenoidal conditions**
- **Cancer of the Larynx (voice box)**

Sinusitis

As we saw in chapter 2 the facial sinuses are the air filled cavities, lined with mucous membrane, which are within the bones surrounding the nose. The two frontal sinuses are just above the eyebrows; the two maxillary sinuses are in the cheekbones; the two ethmoidal sinuses lie between the nasal cavity and the eye sockets and the two sphenoidal sinuses lie behind the nose at the base of the skull.

Sinusitis is an infection of the membranes, and the most commonly affected are those in the cheekbones and between the eyes, and can be both acute (lasting for a couple of weeks) or chronic (lasting for months or even years) in nature.

Sinusitis is caused by a viral infection spreading to the sinuses from the nose, especially when the patient blows his nose vigorously, along the narrow passages that drain mucus from the sinuses into the nose. The sinuses accumulate fluid and mucous which allow bacteria to multiply. It is usually a result of a bacterial infection e.g. Streptococcus pneumniae or Haemophilus influenza that develops as a complication of a viral infection e.g. a common cold (viral rhinitis). Other causes of infection may be from an abscess in an upper tooth; having infected water forced into the sinuses up the nose when jumping into infected water; or as a result of a severe facial injury.

Other predisposing conditions include;

- Allergies
- Cleft palate
- Cystic fibrosis
- Nasal polyps.

When the sinus becomes infected and the amount of mucus produced by the goblet cells of the epithelium of the mucus membrane is considerable, the brush- like filaments called cilia which are attached to epithelium which normally beat and create current to move the mucus towards the drainage passage become 'paralysed'. With the reduction of activity of the cilia the infection in the sinus builds up and has to be treated.

Sinusitis is very common and many people suffer from it after every cold. Once there is an established tendency for it, then recurrence is more likely after every cold. It causes a feeling of fullness in the affected area e.g. pain or tenderness over the forehead, and sometimes an ache. Other symptoms can be a fever, bad breath, ear pressure, upper tooth pain, stuffy nose and loss of sense of smell. Complications can be pus formation causing pain and nasal discharge; orbital cellulitis, osteomyelitis and meningitis are more serious conditions deriving from sinusitis and can lead to major surgery entering either through the nasal passage or the skull.

We have seen that research indicates that glue ear and other types of middle ear infections can be the result of reflux of gastric juices. Acid reflux in the pharynx may also play a part in the development of sinusitis through inflaming nasal mucous which blocks the sinuses. It is also possible that regurgitated gastric acid damages teeth through the loss of dental enamel by chemical process (source: review of studies by Medical College of Wisconsin physicians, USA).

It is possible that sinusitis can be influenced by hormonal changes.

A doctor can use a fibreoptic rhinopharyngoscope to check whether the sinus drainage tubes are blocked and whether the sinuses are inflamed.

Treatment can be undertaken after X-rays have been taken to locate and determine the scale of the disorder (mucosal thickening, air-fluid level and possible complete opacification). CT scan of sinuses is an option - it is more accurate than X-Rays in checking for abnormalities in the sinus linings.

The maxillary sinus can be washed (lavage) and a culture grown to identify the infective bacteria. Oral antibiotic drugs such as Amoxicillin, Erythromycin, Ceftin and Augmentin are used for 10-14 days to combat the infection and these may be changed when the result of the culture is known.

Nose drops or a spray with a decongestant drug or an oral decongestant such as pseudoephedrine restores drainage of the sinuses by reducing the inflammation of the mucous membranes. Steam inhalations, possibly with an oil such as eucalyptus or Olbas helps moisten and remove secretions. Surgical drainage can be carried out if sinusitis persists after other treatments have been followed. This is normally done under general anaesthetic but the author had it done under local anaesthetic and in his case was both unpleasant and a failure.

If there is chronic sinusitis the traditional form of surgery is Functional Endoscopic Sinus Surgery (FESS). This operation can be carried out under local or general anaesthetic and using special instruments small pieces of tissue are removed. The aim of this type of sinus surgery is to remove diseased tissue and allow infected material to drain from the sinus cavities. Unfortunately there can be side effects such as bleeding and loss of smell.
A new laser procedure which has been developed in the USA by Surgical Laser Technologies (SLT) combines laser power with a warm saline water solution to wash away diseased tissue such as polyps. This new technology leads to less bleeding and pain than existing sinus surgery. Recuperation time is shorter being measured in days rather than weeks.

Misdiagnosis of sinusitis

If sinusitis is wrongly diagnosed as rhinitis then if decongestants are used for more than ten days the nose will go into 'rebound' and the medication will cause low-grade damage. This will lead to a congested nasal lining which may need more decongestants and so on. If on the other hand rhinitis is wrongly diagnosed as sinusitis the treatment by antibiotics and decongestants will not calm but actually inflame the sinuses.

Because the pain symptoms are similar, diagnosed sinusitis in fact can often be migraine, tension headaches, jaw or dental problems or malfunction of the trigeminal ganglion in the brain (which is the junction box for the nerves leading to the face) which may be caused by muscle tension initiated by stress.

Rhinitis

Rhinitis is an inflammation of the mucous membrane that lines the nose. There are a number of symptoms which can be suffered in combination - nasal obstruction, nasal discharge, sneezing and facial pressure and/or pain.

There are various types of rhinitis;
- **Viral**
- **Allergic**
- **Vasomotor**
- **Hypertrophic**
- **Atrophic.**

Viral rhinitis

This type is a feature of the common cold and may lead to sinusitis.

Allergic rhinitis

This type is due to an allergy to an airborne substance and is known as 'hay fever'. If caused by pollens from trees, grasses or weeds it is seasonal. Tree pollens are most prevalent in the spring; grass pollen in the summer and weed pollens in the summer and autumn. The worst effects occur on warm and windy days with a high pollen count, especially in flat countryside.

Other triggers such as dusts, moulds, house-dust mites, feathers and pets' hairs and skin scales can cause the condition to occur throughout the year. It most commonly occurs with vasomotor rhinitis (see page 121). The symptoms are a runny nose, sneezing and nasal congestion, and an itching sensation in the nose, throat and eyes. Watery eyes may also be affected by conjunctivitis making them sore and red.

This is a common complaint with up to 10% of the population of the UK being affected. It is more common in those people who suffer from other allergy linked conditions such as asthma or eczema. It is likely to be hereditary, develops before 30 years of age and is predominant in women.

In some people particles of certain harmless substances (allergens) are inhaled and this provokes an exaggerated defence response by the immune system which forms antibodies against them. The allergens also trigger the release of histamine and other chemical substances that cause the inflammation and fluid production in the nose and nasal sinuses.

If the symptoms of the condition do not clear up on their own, treatment usually begins with a skin test to identify the allergen responsible for the condition. Once the trigger allergen is known exposure to it should be minimised. Mild attacks can be treated by decongestant drops or sprays which may take a few days to begin to work on the symptoms. Antihistamine drugs can be taken which reduce the itching, runny nose and nasal congestion; these drugs can cause drowsiness which makes life difficult for those who have to drive, work equipment or take examinations. Corticosteroid drugs are available in nasal spray form.

The drug, sodium cromoglycate inhaled regularly throughout the pollen season may prevent attacks by blocking the allergic response. Long term relief can be gained following desensitization to particular pollen though a course of injections of a gradually increasing dose of the allergen which stimulates the immune system. This will make the immune system less sensitive to the allergen, probably by the production of a 'blocking' antibody. The injections, into the arm, have to be repeated annually for a few years and must be carried out under strict medical conditions to minimise the risks of an anaphylactic shock (severe allergic reaction). The course of injections normally starts before the particular allergen becomes active.

Vasomotor rhinitis

This can be continual or intermittent and the nose becomes too responsive to stimuli. These include pollutants such as tobacco smoke, changes or extremes in temperature, certain foods or medicines or even emotions. It can be common during pregnancy and with those taking combined oral contraceptives and other oestrogen hormone drugs.

Hypertrophic rhinitis

This type has a thickening of the nasal mucous membrane and chronic congestion of the nasal veins which can be caused by repeated nasal infections. It gives a constant stuffy nose and possibly a reduction in the sense of smell. If it is severe there may have to be a surgical removal or shrinkage of the swollen tissue.

Atrophic rhinitis

A wasting of the mucous membrane can be the result of aging, chronic bacterial infections or extensive nasal surgery. Symptoms can include a persistent nasal infection, a discharge which dries to a crust, loss of smell and a nasty odour. Treatment is with antibiotic drugs and sometimes oestrogen drugs.

Snoring

Snoring is noisy breathing through the open mouth during sleep and it is produced by vibrations of the soft palate when air hits the throat directly, the main vibratory tissue is the uvula (the triangular piece of skin which hangs from the soft palate).

Snoring is caused by problems such as a common cold, allergic rhinitis or enlarged adenoids which hinder breathing through the nose because fluid accumulates in the blood vessels around the nasal valves causing the valve openings to narrow. Also the presence of nasal polyp(s) or a small airway.

Snoring is a common condition with serious social (it causes arguments in 15% of UK families, source: BSSAA) and medical implications especially for those who are extremely overweight or have unexplained high blood pressure. In the UK 41% of men and 28% of women are snorers (source: British Snoring and Sleep Apnoea Association (BSSAA)). It progressively worsens in men after 20 years of age and in women after 40 years of age because as we get older the throat muscles relax and fatty tissues build up which combine to close the airway. Many women snore when pregnant because the progesterone hormone may be linked to the condition.

Snoring is more common if the person when sleeping is lying on the back as the lower jaw can drop open. With some people, snoring will alternate with sleep apnoea (a temporary cessation of breathing). Also, the tongue falls backwards into the throat which can narrow the airway and block airflow.

Many factors can affect the natural airflow through the nasal valves at the back of the nostrils. As the valves are only about 0.1 inches wide and surrounded by blood vessels it is easy for them to become constricted with the mouth taking over the job of breathing. If there is a structural condition such as a deviated septum due to a broken nose this will play a part in possibly reducing nasal efficiency.

There are a number of risk factors which may encourage the trumpet voluntary to be heard during the night (not by the snorer but by his/her sleeping partner!), these include;

- **drinking alcohol** - alcohol encourages the muscles in the throat to relax more during sleep so increasing the likelihood of the airway collapsing. About 37% of hardened snorers only snore after they have been drinking alcohol (source: BSSAA)
- **taking drugs** - certain drugs such as tranquillisers can also affect the central nervous system which in turn relaxes the throat muscles
- **obesity** - obesity increases fat deposits in the throat which narrows the air passage. If there is a greater than average amount of fat located around the neck there may not be enough muscle tone to keep the airway open to allow night time normal breathing
- **smoking** - tobacco smoke, including passive smoking, irritates the lining of the nose which leads to a catarrh build up and nasal passage congestion. A smoker is more likely to breathe through the mouth while asleep and the throat is inflamed by the smoke which aggravates the problem. Smokers are twice as likely to snore as non-smokers (source: BSSAA)!

There are a number of treatments which can be considered to reduce snoring. Surgery should be considered as a last resort especially as changes in lifestyle can bring about a dramatic improvement for both the snorer and those affected by the noise which is produced (the loudest snore recorded, peaked at 93 decibels - louder than a passing underground train!).

Treatments include:

- make it uncomfortable for the snorer to lie on the back by sewing something like a squash ball into the pyjamas
- raise the height of the head of the bed to improve body alignment
- reduce contact with allergens such as feathers which trigger allergic rhinitis
- replace pillows with a synthetic filling to deter dust mites
- take appropriate medication
- improve lifestyle - reduce smoking and alcohol, lose weight and take exercise
- wear nasal strips to improve breathing
- wear either a Mandibular Advancement Device (MAD) which holds the lower jaw and tongue forward and assists 'tongue based snorers' or an oral vestibular shield which is designed to keep the mouth closed
- apply an 'Instant Snoring Relief' Spray or use a 'Stopsnore' mouthwash
- use a nasal dilator - especially people with small or collapsing nostrils
- those having to listen to snoring could wear ear plugs
- have a steam inhalation before going to bed and possibly add some essential oils.

The removal of enlarged adenoids can help affected children. There are four surgical procedures which can be undertaken after all simple non-surgical alternatives have been tried and failed. These are;

- Uvulopalatopharyngoplasty (UPPP) - the surgeon trims and tightens throat tissues; the operation is done under a general anaesthetic
- Laser-assisted uvuloplatoplasty (LAUP) - the removal by laser of excess tissue from the soft palate and uvula. The airway is enlarged and vibrations decreased. The operation takes about 30 minutes under local anaesthetic and there may be up to six sessions over a period of time
- Palatal stiffening operations (CAPSO) - this procedure electrically burns the palate causing fibrosis (an overgrowth of scar tissue) with a consequent stiffening of the soft palate with less vibrations, it can also remove a longitudinal strip of mucosa along the soft palate or uvula. The procedure is carried out under local anaesthetic, it may have to be repeated several times for optimum results
- Radio-frequency ablation (Somnoplasty) - this shrinks redundant tissue of the soft palate using a needle attached to a radio frequency generator. This procedure is done under either local or general anaesthetic and repeat treatments may be necessary.

After all these procedures, which are a last resort, there may be some pain; possible side effects and snoring will recur especially if weight is increased in the neck area. The operations are irreversible and may mask the development of sleep apnoea. If UPPP is performed it may affect the possibility of having CPAP oxygen therapy for sleep apnoea.

While the recommended treatment for sleep apnoea is the wearing of an oxygen mask over the face while asleep with air being forced through the airway so that it will not close, this treatment which is called Continuous Positive Airway Pressure (CPAP) can also be effective for snoring.

Sleep apnoea

Sleep apnoea is a condition where there is a temporary cessation of breathing, lasting for 10 seconds or more which occurs during sleep. Sufferers may be excessively sleepy during the day, have poor memory and find difficulty in concentrating. It is potentially dangerous because it can result in hypertension (high blood pressure), heart failure (reduced pumping efficiency), myocardial infarction (heart attack) or stroke. There are three types of sleep apnoea;

- **Obstructive sleep apnoea (OSA)**
- **Central sleep apnoea (CSA)**
- **Mixed sleep apnoea (MSA).**

Obstructive sleep apnoea (OSA)

The same processes of reduced airways which are involved with snoring are found in sleep apnoea but with this condition the airways narrow so much that they close completely. Breathing stops which cuts off the flow of oxygen into the body and also the elimination of carbon dioxide (CO_2) from the blood. The brain detects this rise in CO_2 and briefly wakes you up, normally with a gasp for air; the airways are re-opened and breathing starts again. This process can be repeated many times during the night.

Obstructive sleep apnoea is the most common type of sleep apnoea and while anyone can suffer from it, it is most prevalent in middle- aged men (30 -50 years old) who are overweight and heavy snorers. Possibly 1 in 100 in this age group are affected by the condition.

Central sleep apnoea (CSA)

Breathing stops because the diaphragm and chest muscles temporarily cease working, probably due to a disturbance in the brain's control of breathing. The causes include paralysis of the diaphragm muscles and disturbance in the brainstem. Snoring is not strongly indicated.

Mixed sleep apnoea (MSA)

This is a combined type of sleep apnoea. There can be a pattern of a short period of central sleep apnoea followed by a longer period of obstructive sleep apnoea.

Diagnosis of sleep apnoea

To enable a doctor to recognise sleep apnoea in a patient he/she will take a history which will include the amount of disturbed sleep, excessive daytime sleepiness, loud snoring and any long pauses in breathing which are reported by the patient's partner. If a doctor thinks the diagnosis is probably sleep apnoea then further investigations will be conducted, usually in a sleep laboratory. These will include;

- visual observation of the sleep pattern including laboured breathing and long pauses with sudden arousal from sleep
- measurement of oxygen in the blood and the pulse rate (pulse oximetry)
- Polysomnography - many measures of sleep including eye movement, chin tone, flow of air through the nose and mouth, movement of the chest wall, blood oxygen levels and ECG (electrocardiography)

Treatment of sleep apnoea

We have already seen that there are a number of lifestyle changes which can be made and devices used by snorers before surgery is contemplated. Sufferers from sleep apnoea could also consider following the advice already given to snorers such as reducing alcohol, giving up smoking and having a better lifestyle.

The most common treatment is to wear an oxygen mask over the face while sleeping which is attached to a ventilator machine that keeps the throat open with air forced down the upper airway through the nose. This treatment is called Continuous Positive Airway Pressure (CPAP)

In mild cases, tricyclic antidepressant drugs can be prescribed. The various surgical procedures to help snoring can be applicable for sleep apnoea sufferers. Other possible procedures to remove blockages are; removal of the tonsils (tonsillectomy), removal of the adenoids (adenoidectomy) or the creation of an opening into the windpipe which allows the air to flow to the lungs (tracheostomy).

If sleep apnoea is caused by a jaw deformity the deformity can be corrected surgically by lengthening the jaw bone. This operation has a high success rate.

Headaches

Headaches are one of the most common forms of pain. Usually they are a response to a trigger or combination of triggers but they can occasionally be a symptom of a serious, underlying disorder. The triggers can be internal (hormonal changes, stress or tiredness) or external (weather changes, diet or allergens) or both.

The headache triggers are directed to the hypothalamus which is the part of the brain responsible for regulating hormones, sleep and hunger. If nausea and vomiting are associated with the headache these are initiated by signals sent from the hypothalamus to the part of the upper brain stem which contains the trigeminal nerve. The activation of this nerve whose fibres spread out to cover the whole brain like a helmet is especially important in beginning a migraine.

The headache pain which may be superficial or deep, throbbing or sharp is caused by the swelling of blood vessels in the dura which is the outer covering of the brain. The dura also has pain-sensitive nerve fibres and once the nerves are activated they release compounds that awaken pain receptors which cause the blood vessels to swell even more. It was back in the 17th century that the English physician Thomas Willis suggested that headaches are caused by a rapid increase in the blood flow supply to the brain.

Types of headache

Doctors categorise headaches as;
● self-contained (primary headaches) e.g. a tension headache
● resulting from another illness, condition or injury (secondary headaches) e.g. a hangover after an excess of alcohol or a headache after a bacterial infection.

If a headache is the body's response to a simple trigger such as hunger or a fall in atmospheric pressure then these can improve or clear up with eating or the weather changing in a few hours with little after effect.

Tension headaches caused by a tightening in the muscles of the face, neck or scalp as a result of body imbalance or stress can last for days or weeks and are more inconvenient.
Cluster headaches, which are uncommon, cause intense pain behind one eye and may waken sufferers nightly for a period of weeks or months.
A **migraine** is a severe and incapacitating headache lasting for days or weeks which is usually preceded by visual and/or stomach disturbances.

The causes of headaches

There are a large number of causes of headaches and commonly these include;
● the after effects of drinking alcohol (a 'hangover')
● irregular or lack of meals

- prolonged travel
- poor posture (especially tight neck and shoulder muscles)
- stress or excitement
- Ménière's Disease
- sexual activity - dull ones before orgasm and explosive ones at orgasm
- excessive length of, or lack of, sleep
- certain food triggers including cheese, chocolate and red wine and very cold food e.g. ice cream
- food additives
- incorrect eye glasses and contact lenses
- working in poor light conditions, especially fluorescent lighting
- sinusitis
- toothache
- head injury and concussion
- smoking (especially indicated to cluster headaches)
- cervical osteoarthritis
- overuse of painkillers (analgesics).

Rare causes of headaches include;
- brain tumours
- high blood pressure (hypertension)
- inflammation of arteries in the face, neck and scalp (temporal arteritis)
- ballooning of a blood vessel in the brain (aneurysm)
- increased fluid pressure in the brain.

Treatment of headaches

There are a number of self help steps (which are also covered in chapter 10) which can be carried out and these include;
- identify and avoid a 'trigger' such as excessive alcohol consumption
- try a reduction of sugar intake
- go for a walk outside a stuffy room or office
- have eyes tested regularly and wear correct glasses or contact lenses
- relax in a hot bath or a foot bath (to draw blood away from the head)
- lie down
- stretch and massage back, shoulders, neck, face and scalp muscles
- take mild analgesic tablets
- go to sleep.

Aspirin, paracetemol and ibuprofen are the most common analgesics/painkillers kept in the home. The dose should never be exceeded because an overdose can cause permanent damage to the liver or gastric area.

Cluster headaches, which can get so bad that they are known as suicide headaches, can be treated with oxygen or migraine drugs given intravenously.

If headaches persist without cause and do not respond to self help measures medical aid should be sought. A specialist will conduct physical and neurological tests such as CT scanning, MRI (magnetic resonance imaging), eye tests, neck or sinus X-rays and a lumbar puncture.

There is much current research into the treatment of headaches and predicted results for treatments in the future look promising. It has been reported that the development of a new type of pacemaker primarily for epilepsy could also help chronic headaches, migraine and anxiety. A battery-powered generator the size of a pocket watch is implanted under the skin in the upper chest area; a stimulation electrode links the chest to the neck and is attached to the left vagus nerve. Mild, pre-programmed intermittent electrical pulses are continually delivered to the nerve and it can also be activated manually when headache or migraine symptoms are being experienced or if an epilepsy attack is anticipated. Stimulation of the vagus nerve which originates in the brain and is connected to many parts of the body was found to disrupt abnormal electrical activity in the brain as well as changing chemical neurotransmitters that convey messages across the gaps between the brain nerve cells. Development of this device is at an early stage and is not available to headache or migraine sufferers.

If a headache is caused by trauma such as a sports injury the victim should always seek medical attention at a hospital. Many sports governing bodies such as the Amateur Boxing Association stipulate a minimum time a competitor must wait before competing again after a serious head injury or concussion (temporary unconsciousness).

Migraine
Migraine is a very common condition in the UK with an estimated 10% of the population suffering from it with women being more likely than men to be affected by its symptoms. Usually it starts in the late teens/early twenties with the menopause being another classic time. It can be linked to PMS (premenstrual syndrome) although women on the contraceptive pill can also have it. Young children can suffer, and in the UK each child who suffers from migraine misses an average of four days of school each year (source: the Migraine Trust News, issue No.84). Fortuitously for the over 50s it is extremely rare for the first attack to start after 50.

Many of the symptoms displayed by migraines are also associated with different types of headache and to an extent the two conditions overlap.

While there is no single cause for migraine it does tend to run in families. A number of factors, singly or in combination, may initiate an attack on a susceptible person. The factors may be;
● **stress related** - anger, shock, worry, depression, over-exertion and changes in routine or climate
● **dietary** - many foods including wheat, chocolate, fried food, citrus fruit, red wine, caffeine, cheese and other dairy products, eggs, tea, foods containing monosodium glutamate (E621) and nitrates/nitrites
● **unstable blood sugar levels** (troughs and peaks throughout the day)
● **sensory** - bright lights and loud noises
● **menstruation and the contraceptive pill**
● **possible effects of other drugs or supplements** e.g. Glucosamine
● **TMJ (temperomandibular joint) dysfunction of the jaw** -grinding of teeth, tension of facial muscles and imbalanced bite
● **A defective gene** (in rare cases).

Migraine has been described as a vascular headache and many of the physical phenomena attributed to the development of headaches can be equally applied to migraines. Whilst it has been thought that the pain associated with a headache/migraine is linked to the constriction (narrowing) and dilation (expansion) of blood vessels which have resulted in a headache there has been recent progress in neurological research into the development of a headache/migraine.

Migraine is brought about by chemical changes within the brain which affect the activity of nerves which carry messages about sensations like pain. There is a wave of inactivity (a nerve storm) which passes over the brain prior to an attack. One chemical affected is serotonin, whose levels fall during an attack. Serotonin is associated with constriction of the blood vessels and acts in an area of the brainstem (the 'pain gate') at the top of the spine which prevents us feeling pain.

Normally, the 'pain gate' is kept closed by the brainstem but when the chemical changes the 'gate' is open and the migraine attacks occur. Anxiety opens the gate and relaxation helps close it. Pain is a protective mechanism and a migraine attack could be a warning sign to switch off after stressing the body.

During a migraine attack the trigeminal nerve which directs sensory signals from the face, jaw and top of the forehead floods the brain with pain signals.

Another activity which occurs in the brain during an attack is the filling of the grey matter with oxygen; this triggers chemical reactions which lead to a build up of iron and consequently the brain's ability to block out pain decreases. Migraineurs possibly are more sensitive to pain with each attack.

Types of migraine

There are two types of migraine; **the migraine without aura** (previously called the common migraine) and **the migraine with aura** (previously called the classical migraine).

Migraine without aura/common migraine - This is the type of migraine from which 90% of people ('migraineurs') suffer. The headache pain which slowly develops can mount to a throbbing that is made worse by any slight movement or noise. Often the pain is on one side of the head, starts without warning and is usually linked with nausea, vomiting, cold hands, tremor, dizziness and sensitivity to sound and light. Many sufferers especially children recover after they have been sick. Often social and work arrangements have to be cancelled.

Migraine with aura/classical migraine - This is less common and a headache is preceded by an aura which is a set of internal warning signs which warn the sufferer that an attack is coming, it varies widely in duration between sufferers and generally lasts between a few minutes and one hour. The aura usually stops when a headache starts. This pre-headache stage has been associated with the constriction of blood vessels.

There are three stages to a classical migraine attack;

- the early warning signs (the 'prodomes') and the aura
- the headache and other symptoms phase
- the after effects such as feeling tired (the 'postdromes').

The body prepares its defences against an attack long before the headache starts and it is important that early treatment is taken to control attacks.
Aura and 'prodomes' symptoms can include any, or a combination, of the following;

- visual disturbances - flashing lights, zigzags, coloured stars, blind spots, double vision, blurred vision or loss of vision
- pins and needles, weakness in arms, hands, legs or feet usually on one side and possible temporary paralysis
- changes in understanding people, the world and objects
- slurred speech
- yawning and lassitude
- mood changes
- premonitions
- enhanced sense of smell e.g. paint or perfume
- nasty taste in the mouth.

During the acute phase of the attack most sufferers just want to lie or sit quietly in a darkened room. Conversely, people with mild attacks may want to stay active. As well as the headache and sickness/nausea (which indicates that the gastrointestinal tract is involved), other symptoms can include;

- sensitivity to light
- diarrhoea
- frequent urination or fluid retention
- feeling very hot or very cold
- increased sensitivity to sounds or smells
- speech problems
- lethargy.

After the attack has ceased (the 'postdromal' stage) most sufferers feel worn out and exhausted and not able to do much for up to a few days. Others can have a sense of wellbeing and a state of exhilaration; these people eschew drug therapy and allow the attack to take its natural course.

A doctor can usually make a diagnosis from the patient's history and a physical examination. Special tests are not usually necessary unless there are persistent symptoms, the nature of the headaches change or become more severe, in this scenario a neurological examination is carried out to exclude the possibility of an underlying serious condition.

If the attacks are less frequent than one a month then only the acute attacks need treating. If they are more frequent then preventative treatment may be needed as well. A diary should be kept to record activities which may be triggering attacks.

The simplest treatment is by administering aspirin or paracetemol together with an antemetic drug (often as a suppository). If this medication is not successful then either sumatriptan, which acts on the blood vessels in and around the brain, or ergotamine may be prescribed. Some ergotamine preparations can help prevent an attack if taken early enough before the headache starts.

If excessively sensitive nerve cells are the problem, sumatriptan copies the action of serotonin, which is a neurotransmitter, one of whose actions is to regulate pain and mood. The drug prevents the nerve endings in the dura of the brain from releasing stimulatory protein - the result is no pain.

A new class of drug, the triptans, e.g. 'Relpax', gives sufferers great relief especially if taken early. They usually give temporary relief and have certain side effects especially for those at risk from stroke or heart disease. As well as blocking serotonin pathways triptans also block one of the stimulatory proteins (CGRP) produced in the dura's nerve endings with a consequent reduction in pain. The drug can be administered both intravenously and in tablet form. A new triptan drug 'Zomig' is available in the form of a nasal spray which enters the bloodstream in five minutes and reduces pain within fifteen minutes. Another sumatriptan nasal spray called 'Imigran' has been approved for use on adolescents (12 -17 years) in most of Europe including the UK.

Falling levels of the hormone oestrogen in the lead up to menstruation can trigger an attack. However, many women on hormone replacement therapy (HRT) with high levels of the hormone also experience migraine with aura. Either way the hypothalamus, which is the part of the brain responsible for controlling the menstrual cycle, plays an important part in migraines.

It is thought that if a migraine is not treated early then a mechanism occurs in the central nervous system which makes traditional medication less effective.

Most sufferers find that they recover more quickly if they lie undisturbed in either a prone or semi upright position in a darkened room, often with a damp flannel over the eyes.

If attacks are more frequent than one a month beta-blocker and calcium channel blocker drugs may be prescribed. Calcium channel blockers prevent the movement of calcium across the membrane which lines muscle cells which is an integral part of muscle contraction. Other forms of drug can be prescribed such as anti-depressants, non-steroidal anti-inflammatories and prostaglandin (hormonal) inhibitors. An effective treatment programme is usually found and specialist migraine clinics can give advice.

An unusual side effect of Botox injections which are designed to temporarily eliminate facial wrinkles is that for many sufferers headaches seem to be reduced.

If the migraines are being caused by jaw (TMJ) problems then a dentist can take an impression of the teeth and construct a brace which can be worn to stop the clenching of teeth and reduce tension in the facial muscles so reducing pain.

There are a number of events or conditions which are linked with migraines and these include;

- **abdominal migraine** - pain, nausea and vomiting in migraine sufferers
- **epileptic migraine** - concurrence of epilepsy and migraine
- **facioplegic migraine** - unilateral and transient palsy occurring in a migraine attack
- **hemiplegic migraine** - recurrent episodes of hemiplegia (weakness or paralysis on one side) during a migraine attack
- **ophthalmic migraine** - any of many visual symptoms during an attack
- **ophthalmoplegic migraine** - paralysis of a cranial ocular nerve

Motion Sickness

Many forms of transport have the ability to make certain people ill; car sickness, sea sickness, air sickness, space sickness, travel sickness and simulator sickness. Many different physical and emotional stimuli can lead to a victim suffering a progression of symptoms from epigastric discomfort/ 'stomach awareness', pallor and sweating through to debilitating nausea and vomiting. Feelings of lethargy, tiredness and headaches are other common symptoms. Hyperventilation is sometimes observed.

The development of sickness can range from a few minutes to a few hours and there are also the after effects of vertigo and dizziness. Sometimes vomiting happens after cessation of movement. If exposure to motion continues for several days there can be a cyclical pattern of the nausea and vomiting waxing and waning. Motion brings misery to people who do not vomit.

Sea sickness was known in ancient times by sailors ('naus' is a Greek word for ship and is the root for nausea meaning 'an inclination to vomit'); with the coming of other forms of travel on land and in the air the term changed to travel sickness; with the viewing of certain films and body oscillation on fairground and playground rides the name of the syndrome changed to motion sickness.

The main players in the cause of motion sickness are the inner ear's vestibular (balance and motion centre) and the eye's visual sensory systems. The vestibular system is found in both ears and comprise the 3 fluid filled semicircular canals which are responsible for sensing head rotational movements and the utricle and saccule balance components of the vestibule. Nerve fibres from these areas connect to the brain's cerebellum and also to other nerve nuclei including those involved with the control of eye movements.

The processes of the semicircular canals and the parts of the vestibule are extremely complex and suffice to say that while some theorists have pointed to the canals being involved with motion sickness, others think it is the otoliths which are located in the vestibule's utricle and saccule. It is generally now accepted that both systems are involved when the problem arises with their signals indicating different motions of the head.

The visual system can also provoke motion sickness and this can be demonstrated when watching films conveying movement. It is sometimes only necessary to watch a film through wide view and the most provocative imply that the viewer is in motion. When the eyes are closed motion sickness can be stimulated.

Another factor to be considered in the question of motion sickness is the involvement of the somatosensory/somatic system which is distributed throughout the body and which responds to changes in force and displacement and senses body movements and applied force. It is not always apparent which of the sensory systems will first detect the motion which causes the sickness.

There are also many psychological factors involved with the susceptibility of individuals to motion sickness. These include the receptiveness, adaptability and retentiveness of individuals to their internal model of motion. Some studies (Kottenhoff and Lindahl, 1960) have suggested that introverts are more susceptible to motion sickness; there is a positive correlation between neuroticism and motion sickness susceptibility (Guedry and Ambler, 1972; Lentz and Collins, 1977).
Studies have shown that susceptibility is highest between 2 and 12 years of age and a gradual decline in susceptibility occurs throughout life. Women are more prone than men and this may be due to anatomical or hormonal differences. Schwab (1954) reported that women are more likely to be sick during menstruation and Reason (1957) suggested that motion sickness is more common during pregnancy. Several studies have shown that there is an increased susceptibility to motion sickness in those children suffering from migraine (e.g. Barabas et al., 1983).

There are a number of measures to prevent motion sickness including;
- tasks should be designed to require the minimum of head and eye movements
- good environmental conditions (e.g. heating and ventilation)
- passengers should be located where oscillation is least e.g. in the centre of a ship
- entertainment should not require head or eye movement
- environments should be avoided where there are frequent changes in speed and direction
- it may be beneficial to lie down on the back with the head supported
- the head should be fixed and supported on a headrest
- if sickness is anticipated, make contingency arrangements (possibly a sick bag) before symptoms appear and then forget about them
- light consumption of food and drink prior to a journey and do not eat during a journey if head movements can cause a problem
- engage in mental or physical activities that do not need repeated head or eye movements e.g. singing

132

- drugs may have detrimental side effects e.g. drowsiness - especially important for drivers
- do not allow eyes to follow movement of nearby objects; especially those in motion e.g. other vehicles
- try 'alternative' remedies such as root ginger and homeopathic substances such as Rhus Tox and Tabacum which should be taken under the direction of a qualified Homeopath
- wear an acupressure strap on the Nei-Kuan acupressure meridian point just above the wrist
- try cognitive counselling and biofeedback therapy procedures.

Nasal Polyps

A polyp is a growth which projects, usually on a stalk from the mucous membrane of the nasal passage. Polyps can be found in other parts of the body including the cervix, intestine and larynx.

They can be treated homeopathically but usually have to be removed surgically if they cause symptoms such as restricted breathing or difficulty in speaking. Some types of polyp can cause cancer and have to be removed even if there are no symptoms. Often a nasal polyp can grow into the size of a grape, a polyp can regrow and surgery has to be repeated. If there are repeated nasal operations there is a risk of atrophic rhinitis occurring.

Polyps may give divers problems. When descending, a nasal polyp may be pressed against the entrance to the maxillary antrum (cavity) blocking it and giving pain. On ascending, a polyp in the antrum may do the same on the other side. Divers with polyps must not dive or go under pressure.

Facial neuralgia

Neuralgia is a pain caused by damage to or irritation of a nerve. The pain can be severe or is felt shooting along the affected nerve. As well as **Trigeminal Neuralgia (TN)** which is a disorder of the trigeminal cranial nerve there are other syndromes which are very similar to TN but have specific unique features, these include;

- **post-herpetic (shingles) neuralgia**
- **atypical facial pain (ATFP)**
- **the result of Multiple Sclerosis (MS)**
- **other neuralgias - Glossopharyngeal; Geniculate; Vegal and Superior Laryngeal neuralgia and Occipital neuralgia**
- **dental disorders.**

Trigeminal Neuralgia (TN)

TN is also known as Tic Douloureux ('painful spasm' - a description given by 18th century French surgeon Nicolaus Andre) and is very rare, affecting 150 per million people per year; the condition was written up by Aretaeus in the first century A.D.

There are two trigeminal nerves, one on the right side of the head; the other on the left side. It is the fifth cranial nerve and has three distinct branches (V1, V2 and V3) on each side.

THE TRIGEMINAL NERVE

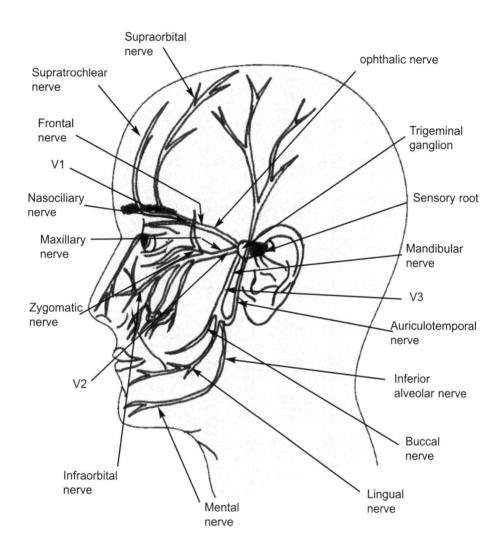

V1 = Opthalmic branch
V2 = Maxillary branch
V3 = Mandibular branch

V1 (Opthalmic) is a sensory nerve affecting the eye, forehead and nose

V2 (Maxillary) is a sensory nerve affecting the upper teeth, gums and lip, the cheek, lower eyelid and the side of the nose

V3 (Mandibular) is a sensory nerve affecting the lower teeth, gums and lip; it is also a motor nerve affecting the jaw.

Sensory nerves: transmit pressure, touch, pain and temperature signals to the brain.

Motor nerves: control movement stimulated by the brain.

TN pain can be described as sudden, shooting or stabbing which lasts for several seconds over the course of the day. It is usually unilateral but can be on both sides of the face (bilateral). The pain is triggered by touching specific points on the face during the actions of talking, eating or shaving. The triggers vary between people and the pain may last for days, weeks or months and then be in remission and disappear for months or years.

There are many causes of TN and these include;
- pressure of a blood vessel on the root of a trigeminal nerve
- destruction of the myelin sheath (demyelinisation), which protect nerve fibres, faster than it can be regenerated with scarring that disrupts nerve signals, TN is rarely the first symptom of Multiple Sclerosis but typically appears in the advanced stage of MS
- nerve damage caused by dental or surgical procedures; facial injury or infection
- pressure of a tumour on the nerve (rare)
- no clear cause
- possible inheritance of TN

After a medical examination and case history have been taken a number of advanced test options are available and these include CT scan, MRI and high definition angiography (MRTA). A number of drugs including carbamazepine or treptal can be used alone or in combination. If drugs fail, surgery can be considered such as Microvascular Depression (MVD).

Atypical Facial Pain (ATFP) syndrome

ATFP syndrome covers a wide number of facial pain problems with different causes and similar symptoms. The pain is described as burning, aching or cramping occurring on one side only in the area of the trigeminal nerve but extending into the upper neck or back of the scalp. It is not as severe as with trigeminal neuralgia (TN) but is continuous with few remission periods. Some patients have symptoms associated with both ATFP and TN.

There are many causes of ATFP including;
- infection of the teeth or sinuses
- nerve damage caused by low grade infectious and inflammatory processes over a long period
- vascular decompression of the trigeminal nerve in the same area as that which causes TN
- dental or other trauma.

The syndrome often needs many dental and medical checks before it is diagnosed successfully. MRI and CT scans often concentrate on the skull base. Drug treatment is usually more successful then surgery. Drugs can include amitriptyline or neurontin. Pain relief may be brought about by using hot and cold compresses, acupuncture, biofeedback or a dental splint.

Herpes and Post herpetic Neuralgia

Post herpetic Neuralgia is a chronic condition which can develop in mainly older people whose immune system has been affected by an attack of shingles (herpes zoster virus). While sufferers of shingles which can attack the limbs or torso as well as the face (trigeminal ganglia shingles) have pain for about one month some sufferers of Post herpetic Neuralgia (2%- 3%) can have chronic pain for more than one year.

While the treatment of shingles is normally a combination of antiviral and analgesic medication with possible L-Lysine supplements and a high protein diet, post herpetic neuralgia is treated with a tricyclic anti-depressant such as amitriptyline in conjunction with an anticonvulsant such as carbamazepine. In the United States opioid therapy can be prescribed. Creams for localised affected areas have to be administered carefully as they may irritate the eye and the skin around the eye.

Glossopharyngeal Neuralgia

This is a deep stabbing pain in one side of the throat, near the tonsil area and possibly extending into the ear, jaw or upper lateral neck. This pain is caused by a compression of the Glossopharyngeal nerve and is often triggered by swallowing, talking, or clearing the throat (not chewing or touching the face).

Although attacks are similar to TN it is much less common (about 1:100). The condition can be treated with drugs or then by surgery in appropriate cases.

Geniculate Neuralgia

Geniculate neuralgia is another name for Nervus intermedius neuralgia. This is a very uncommon condition and is a disturbance of cranial facial nerve VII. There is a stabbing pain similar to an electric shock deep in the ear which can be triggered by a non-noxious stimulation of the inner ear canal or can follow swallowing or talking. There is no residual pain between attacks.

This syndrome is always unilateral and during attacks the symptoms can be salivation, bitter taste, tinnitus or vertigo. There may also be an irritation of the vestibulocochlear cranial nerve VIII.

The primary cause of this neuralgia is compression of the nerve. It can also be caused by the herpes zoster virus, if this is the case there is a vesicular eruption on the ear drum and external ear canal with pain after one to two days. The pain is constant and burning and is different to the intermittent stabbing pain of nervus intermedius tic.

Treatment is either by medication similar to that for trigeminal neuralgia. If this is not successful anaesthetics can be injected into the Glossopharyngeal or Trigeminal nerve to ascertain that it is the nervus intermedius which is the cause. Surgery is an option, including Gamma Knife surgery.

Vegal and Superior Laryngeal Neuralgia

This rare neuralgia affects the two sensory branches of the vagus nerve - the auricular branch and the superior laryngeal nerve - and is caused by a compression of the upper fibres of the vagal nerve when they leave the brain stem.

The pain trigger zone is in the larynx and attacks are initiated by talking, swallowing, yawning or coughing. If other sections of the vagus nerve are involved there may be hiccups, excessive salivation or inspiratory stridor (abnormal in breath sound). Shock - like pain can be felt in the third cartilage, jaw and ear. It is similar to Trigeminal neuralgia except in its location.

The superior laryngeal nerve can be anesthetised and if drug medication (similar to that for Trigeminal Neuralgia) is not successful then surgery is an option, surgery is usually successful.

Occipital Neuralgia

Occipital neuralgia is another uncommon syndrome. It is characterized by a continuous aching or throbbing pain in the back of the head and in the sub occipital region. The pain is not triggered but pressure over the occipital nerves can exacerbate it. It is different to muscle tension headache pain in this area.

There are several causes including; trauma to the greater or lesser occipital nerves, compression of these nerves or upper cervical roots by arthritic changes in the spine or tumours affecting the 2nd and 3rd cervical dorsal roots. Often, emotional or physical tension is a factor to be taken into account.

Positive diagnosis is determined by neurological tests. Roentgenography/X-rays (after Wilhelm Conrad Roentgen who discovered X-rays in 1895) and CT scans can help with diagnosis.

Treatment regime varies; if it is structural the cause is treated. If it is symptomatic and the pain is similar to Trigeminal neuralgia anticonvulsants can be tried. If the pain resembles atypical facial pain a tricyclic antidepressant and a phenathiazine combination can be used. Nerve blocks, local anaesthetics and steroids are options. Surgery is not necessary for the vast majority of patients.

Dental disorders

There are a number of different titles for neuralgia which has possibly been induced by dental treatment e.g. Roberts bone cavity, trigger bone cavity, Ratner bone cavities, interference field and most commonly NICO (Neuralgia-Inducing Cavitational Osteonecrosis).

NICO is thought to cause referred pain and neuralgia -like symptoms to other parts of the face, intraoral cavity and head from the primary site of the jaw. Pain is constant, burning and cramping like ATFP and the trigger points over the jaw will be painful if pressed. NICO starts after dental procedures such as tooth extraction, jaw surgery or crown preparation. It is thought that small areas of bone become infected and die; this process is not indicated on an X-ray. There could be established low-grade infection and it is possible that blood vessels in the area are injured with poor circulation and consequent bone death.

The only treatment for NICO is jawbone curettage where the jawbone is opened, the affected part drilled out, a biopsy done to confirm the presence of infection or inflammation and a possible packing of a bone cavity with antibiotics e.g. terramycin (a brand name for oxytetracycline) . A course of antibiotics may also be prescribed. This operation is not done routinely.

This syndrome is quite controversial and NICO is not considered by some dentists and medical practitioners to be either the cause of Trigeminal neuralgia or even the condition to be a disorder. Some dentists think that NICO is the cause of many facial pain syndromes and that curettage can cure the painful conditions. In this second group some members think that root canal and mercury fillings are partly responsible for NICO.

Bell's palsy

Bell's palsy is a condition in which one side of the face becomes paralysed, it is usually temporary and most cases (80%) begin to get better without treatment within three weeks and an early improvement is an indication that there will be a complete recovery. It is named after Sir Charles Bell a 19th century Scottish physician and anatomist who first linked the condition to a problem with the 7th (VII) cranial nerve which is also known as the facial nerve and comprises 7,000 nerve fibres.

The facial paralysis usually comes on suddenly, often in a few hours or overnight, however in some cases its onset may be gradual. It has no apparent cause such as an injury. In the UK, 1 in 60/70 people will be affected at some time. Most cases are in people over 40 years of age; men and women are equally affected although pregnancy brings a threefold risk to women. About 10% of people who suffer an attack, especially women when they become pregnant, will be affected again in the future. Usually a second attack affects the opposite side of the face.

While the exact cause of this socially distressing condition is not known it is thought that a viral infection of the facial nerve is often involved. The herpes simplex virus, which also causes cold sores around the mouth, may lie dormant in the facial nerve and cause inflammation when it is active. Mumps, HIV and rubella may also be triggers. Bacterial infections like Lyme's disease or tuberculosis can cause inflammation and swelling of the facial nerve that causes Bell's Palsy. A tumour, skull fracture or neurological conditions caused by chronic diseases are also factors in causing Bell's Palsy. Diabetes, traumatic head injury and flu/common cold may increase the risk and it may also be a hereditary problem.

The author recently met a lovely older lady whose Bell's palsy was thought to have been caused by an attack of shingles (Herpes zoster virus) in the ear. She demonstrated all the classic symptoms of Bell's palsy and had her affected eye protected by wearing a patch.

There are a number of symptoms, the main ones being paralysis/weakness on one side of the face, a sagging eyebrow and difficulty in closing the eye. Other symptoms can include;

- face numbness
- dry mouth
- difficulty of speech
- loss of taste in the front part of the tongue
- dryness/watering of the affected eye and a turned out lower eyelid
- dribbling when drinking or after cleaning teeth
- ear pain; especially below the ear
- intolerance to loud noise on the affected side.

In a few cases, new muscle fibres that grow back after the paralysis connect to the wrong facial muscle - this results in lasting damage and can cause any of the following (singly or in combination);

- facial spasms
- twitching
- blinking when trying to smile
- involuntary movement of the corners of the mouth when closing the eyes
- formation of false 'crocodile' tears at the same time as saliva.

Usually a doctor can identify Bell's palsy by examining the condition of the face and listening to the recounted symptoms. When there is doubt an EMG (electromyography) test can measure the electrical activity of the facial muscles. If there is no improvement after three weeks imaging tests such as X-ray or MRI will help to eliminate other causes of paralysis.

Even though the condition usually improves by itself a course of steroids can be started within the first 24 hours. Acyclovir, an antiviral drug, may also be prescribed - there is little evidence that these treatments are effective.

Self help may stimulate recovery including massaging the face using a moisturiser; exercising the facial muscles in front of a mirror and applying gentle heat to reduce pain e.g. with the use of a microwaveable wheat bag.

With Bell's palsy there is a problem in closing the affected eyelid. The following can help prevent the surface of the eyeball drying out;

- using a finger (not the thumb), regularly close the eyelid to moisten the eye ball
- wear protective glasses to guard against dust or other foreign bodies
- tape the eye closed whilst sleeping
- apply suitable 'eye drops' to keep the eyeball moist - ask a pharmacist for advice

- a small dose of Botox (botulinum toxin) can be injected into the upper eyelid - this causes it to temporarily droop so protecting the eye
- faradic current stimulation avoiding the eye area
- complementary therapies include massage, aromatherapy (use oils which are recommended for neuralgia) reflexology, acupuncture, homeopathy, Traditional Chinese Medicine and ear candles.

If people suffer with long term paralysis there are several treatment options including;
- 'facial retraining' physical therapy may be implemented
- tarsorrhaphy, a surgical technique, which narrows the space between the eye lids may improve eye closure
- further use of steroid drugs
- the hormone ACTH (adrenocorticotrophic hormone) which stimulates the body's own steroid production (in the cortex of the adrenal glands)
- a gold weight may be fitted into the upper affected eyelid to help keep the eye lid closed (it will still open properly)
- surgery to relieve pressure on the facial nerve - this is rarely recommended
- plastic surgery to improve permanent facial drooping

Other conditions which cause facial paralysis

There are several other conditions which can result in facial paralysis;
- pressure on the facial nerve - e.g. a tumour
- bacterial infections such as Lyme disease which is spread by tics
- Sarcoidosis - a rare condition of the autoimmune system which mainly affects young adults
- disorders which affect the immune system such as HIV/AIDS
- facial wounds.

The diagnosis and treatment of these causes of facial paralysis is obviously diverse and is not in the scope of this book. Suitable information can be found elsewhere.

Common colds and influenza (the 'flu')

The Common Cold

A cold is a viral infection which causes inflammation of the mucous membranes which line the nose and throat. This leads to a stuffy, runny nose and possibly a sore throat, headache and other miserable side effects for the sufferer.

There are almost 200 viruses which can cause colds; the most common belong to either the rhinoviruses (110 types), which are most active in early autumn/spring/ summer, or the coronaviruses groups (only 4 of 30 strains affect humans), which are most active in the winter and early spring. Cold viruses only live in the noses of humans, chimpanzees and other higher primates- not in other animals.

The viruses grow best at temperatures of 33°C/91°F - the temperature of the human nasal mucosa and they survive better when humidity is low in the colder months of the year. Cold weather may also make the lining of the nasal passages drier and more vulnerable to viral infection.

Colds can be contracted in several ways;
- by inhaling virus-containing droplets which have been sneezed or coughed into the atmosphere
- by rubbing the eyes or nose with fingers which have picked up a virus by bodily contact (usually hands)
- by handling contaminated items such as tea towels or hand towels.

Most people can contract a cold but the incidence is highest among young children because they have not developed immunity to the many viruses to which they are exposed and which they pass to each other mainly at school. Older people have developed immunity to the different viruses. Colds are more common in the winter when people are crowded together indoors or on trains or buses. Many people catch a cold on aeroplanes or in air conditioned premises when they breathe in contaminated recycled air or other people's virus droplets. It has been estimated that in the United States there are almost one billion colds each year. In 1996, 62 million colds in the USA required either medical attention or resulted in restricted activity and 22 million days were lost from school (US National Center for Health Statistics (NCHS)).

How do viruses work?

Viruses cause infections by overcoming the body's defence mechanisms. Mucus, the first line of defence, is produced in the membranes of the nose and throat to trap inward materials such as pollen, dust, bacteria and viruses. When a virus penetrates the mucus and enters a cell it uses its protein-making machinery to manufacture new viruses which attack surrounding cells.

How does the body fight back?

Cold symptoms are probably the result of the immune system fighting back against the invading virus. The affected cells in the nose send out signals that bring specialised white blood cells to the site of infection, these blood cells emit a number of immune system chemicals e.g. kinins, histamine, interleukins and prostaglandins. The chemicals cause swelling and inflammation of the mucus membrane; leakage of proteins and fluid from capillaries and lymph vessels and increased production of mucus. Inflammatory mediators also activate sneeze and cough reflexes and stimulate nerve pain. It is interesting that 25% of people with the cold virus infection do not develop any symptoms and these people recover from the infection as well as those who have the symptoms.

Symptoms of a 'common cold'

'Head colds' are nose and throat infections. Symptoms are a tickle in the throat, watery eyes, sneezing and a moist nasal discharge. The discharge may become infected and the colour changes to yellow or green. The symptoms often worsen and include;
- slight fever
- sore throat
- a productive wet or non-productive dry cough
- aching muscles or bones throughout the body or localised
- headache
- lethargy
- chills
- swollen lymph glands.

Infection can spread and can cause any of the following;
- laryngitis and croakiness or loss of voice
- tracheitis - inflammation of the trachea/windpipe
- acute bronchitis
- sinusitis
- Otitis media - inflammation of the middle ear
- aggravation of existing respiratory disorders such as asthma, chronic bronchitis or chronic ear infections
- reactivation of dormant herpes simplex virus - causing cold sores.

Most colds clear up within about seven days. A doctor should be consulted in the following circumstances;
- the cold does not clear up
- the infection has spread beyond the nose or throat
- a chronic chest infection or ear disorder has been aggravated

Most colds will clear up without treatment. Antibiotics do not kill viruses and it is only if a secondary bacterial infection develops that a course of antibiotic drugs is followed. Researchers are looking at the future use of the drug Interferon or the use of synthetic allergens which will stimulate the immune system to produce antibodies. The difficulty in developing a cold vaccine is that there are so many different cold viruses each of which has its own antigens which lead to the formation of antibodies (protective proteins) by the body. The antigens are often mutating and for this reason the influenza vaccine has to be altered each year to take account of changes in the influenza viruses which have the same basic mechanism as cold viruses.

Many people try to stay out of drafts, avoid dampness and consume large quantities of vitamin C in the form of supplements or foods such as citrus fruit. Unfortunately there has been no conclusive data to support the premise that vitamin C will prevent a cold, it may however reduce the severity or duration of symptoms.

Over the counter cold remedies include a mild analgesic (painkiller) drug such as aspirin or paracetemol which are designed to help relieve aches and pains. Other common ingredients include antihistamine and decongestant drugs which help to reduce nasal congestion and caffeine which is a mild stimulant.

In the USA the National Institute of Allergy and Infectious Diseases (NIAID) has found that exposure to cold weather, getting chilled or overheated had little or no effect on the development or severity of a cold. Susceptibility is not linked to exercise, diet, enlarged tonsils or adenoids. Conversely, psychological stress, allergic disorders affecting the nasal passages or throat, and menstrual cycles did affect people's susceptibility to catch a cold.

Influenza (The 'flu')

Influenza is a viral infection of the respiratory tract that causes fever, headache, muscle ache and weakness. It is spread by virus infected droplets which are coughed or sneezed in the air. Outbreaks, which can develop into epidemics, occur mainly in the winter and spread rapidly in schools and in places which elderly people use. The symptoms of flu vary depending on the type of flu virus involved.

There are three main types of flu virus - A, B, C. Whilst anyone who is affected by any of these separate strains of virus builds up antibodies (proteins produced by the immune system) that provide immunity against that particular strain there is no defence against a different strain or new strains of A and B virus which may be produced and which may be able to overcome the built up immunity.

Type B virus is fairly stable but can change enough to overcome resistance e.g. Hong Kong flu (2001); type A virus is highly unstable and new strains form constantly all over the world - these are the pandemic (worldwide) strains e.g. Spanish flu (1918), Asian flu (1957) Hong Kong flu (1968), Moscow and New Caledonia flus (1999).
The 'Spanish flu' of 1918-1919 killed more people worldwide (20 - 40 million) than either World War I or the Bubonic Plague of 1347 - 1351 and its victims were mainly young adults rather that the old and children.

The symptoms of virus types A and B, of which type A is more debilitating, are chills, fever, headache, muscular aches, loss of appetite and tiredness.

Type C causes a mild illness which is indistinguishable from a cold.

After the initial flu symptoms there can be the onset of other symptoms such as a cough, chest pain, sore throat and a runny nose. After a couple of the days the fever should go and after five days all the symptoms should disappear. There may be some residual respiratory symptoms and possibly a feeling of weakness and/or depression which should be gone after two weeks.

With a type B virus the biggest problem is secondary bacterial infection especially in older people and if they suffer from lung or heart problems they may develop fatal bronchitis, bronchiolitis or pneumonia.

Anti-flu vaccines, containing killed strains of types A and B virus in circulation, have been developed but as these are short lived in their efficiency their administration has to be repeated each year just before the start of the flu season. It is necessary to repeat the 'flu jabs' because the vaccines have to be modified to combat changes in the structure of the viruses which are constantly evolving. The priority for vaccination (in October) should be;

- people over 65 as their immune system is weakened with age and consequently they are more likely to develop serious complications such as pneumonia
- people with chronic disorders of the pulmonary or cardiovascular systems
- those with diabetes, kidney or liver disease or chronic anaemia

- those with chronic malignant conditions such as leukaemia and lymphoma
- those with blood disorders such as sickle cell disease
- individuals undergoing chemotherapy or radiation treatment for cancer
- recipients of organ transplants under medication to prevent rejection
- those on high levels of corticosteroids to control conditions such as rheumatoid arthritis, severe psoriasis and endocrine disorders.

Others who should be high in priority include women in the second and third trimester of pregnancy during the flu season and all healthcare personnel.

People with egg allergies and who have had a previous vaccine-associated allergic reaction should avoid immunisation.

Unless an attack is mild a person with flu should stay in bed in a warm, well ventilated room. Painkillers can be taken to reduce fever and ease aching limbs and muscles. Warm liquids can ease a sore throat and water drunk to reduce dehydration. Steam inhalations possibly with an added essential oil e.g. eucalyptus has a soothing effect on the lungs and will help to keep the airways clear. If sufferers are at risk e.g. old people, a doctor should be called as soon as possible and an antiviral drug like amantadine given which reduces the symptoms if administered in the first 24 hours of onset of symptoms. Antibiotics can combat a secondary bacterial infection.

Once the fever has abated the patient can get out of bed, rest and build up strength. Obviously with both colds and flu, care has to be taken not to infect others.

A research team at Imperial College, London led by Dr Tracy Hussell has had encouraging results from the trials of a new drug named OX40: Ig. This drug is designed to damp down the body's response to a flu virus. The exaggerated defence response includes nasal congestion, breathing difficulties and weight loss. The response produces inflammatory molecules which lead to a cytokine storm whereby too many cells block airways and prevent efficient transfer of oxygen into the bloodstream. OX40: Ig has been identified as a protein which could control the activity of T-cells (an important type of white blood cell). The experiments were conducted on mice with influenza 'A' strain; those with the drug were much healthier than those without the drug.

Laryngitis

Laryngitis is inflammation of the larynx and nearby structures. The larynx, which is commonly called the 'Adam's apple', is the voice box chamber located at the top of the airway to the lungs (the windpipe and trachea) and stretched across it are the membrane folds known as the vocal cords. When air passes over the vocal cords they vibrate to produce sound. The tongue, lips and teeth all play a part in turning sound into speech. When the area, especially the vocal cords, is swollen and irritated the voice becomes hoarse, muted or lost completely and there may occasionally be an obstruction of the airway.

Causes of laryngitis

A viral or bacterial infection is the most common acute cause of laryngitis. Acute cases normally last for a few days. Whilst a common cold could have laryngitis as one of its symptoms, along with sore throat, cough, sneezing, runny cold, fever, tiredness etc, it may be the only symptom.

Other causes of **acute laryngitis** include;
●   bronchitis or pneumonia
●   an upper respiratory infection - which is a self limiting condition
●   an allergy to an inhaled substance such as pollen, dust or spores, which can lead to sneezing, wheezing, congestion and itchy eyes/throat.

There can also be **chronic laryngitis** which persists for a longer period and this can be caused by;
●   excessive use of the voice - cheering for a successful rugby team or chanting at a demonstration
●   a malignant tumour, laryngeal polyp or a laryngeal paralysis e.g. Horner syndrome (a symptom of which is a drooping eyelid on one side) - these are rare causes
●   violent coughing
●   irritation due to tobacco smoke - passive or self inflicted
●   exposure to fumes
●   damage during surgery.

There are several forms of laryngitis which affect children and which can lead to significant or fatal respiratory obstruction, including croup (major symptoms being hoarseness, a grunting noise during breathing and a barking cough) and epiglottitis (inflammation of the epiglottis flap which closes the larynx during swallowing).

Treatment of laryngitis

An examination by a medical practitioner, including listening to the voice, will confirm the condition as laryngitis. A patient, especially a smoker, who has persistent hoarseness, may have to see a specialist for tests on the throat and upper airway. Diagnostic tests can check for signs of cancer of the larynx, which represents about 2% of all cancers, which can be cured if treated at an early stage.

As most laryngitis is viral, generally antibiotics treatment is not indicated. 'Silence is golden' so resting the voice completely will help the voice and reduce inflammation of the vocal cords. A sufferer should also;
●   rest in bed
●   avoid alcohol and tobacco
●   keep the throat lining moist with humidifiers (either use a room humidifier or put wet towels over radiators)
●   inhale warm steam (cover a head with a towel and lean over a bowl of boiling water) - take safety precautions
●   drink lots of fluids, especially warm drinks (chicken soup is a tried remedy).

Decongestants and analgesics, such as paracetemol, may help reduce fever and relieve pain. Doctors will be most concerned if the symptoms do not subside within four - five days, if sputum /phlegm is produced or if the hoarseness lasts for several weeks. If it is a bacterial infection antibiotics drugs will be prescribed.

If a child with croup struggles for breath and turns blue medical help should be sought immediately. If the child is taken to hospital he/she may be given humidified oxygen in a tent. If the throat is seriously obstructed, a breathing tube may be passed down the throat or a tracheostomy operation carried out to insert a tube bypassing the obstruction. Either tube is removed after a couple of days and complete recovery takes place within a few more days.

Tonsillitis

Tonsillitis is an acute infection of the tonsils with the Streptococcus bacterium being the most common infecting organism. Other organisms include Haemophilus influenzae and Streptococcus pyogenes. Tonsillitis is most prevalent among   children under nine although it can occur in juveniles and adolescents. Acute tonsillitis may become chronic.

Symptoms of tonsillitis

There are a number of symptoms which include;
- a sore throat and difficulty in swallowing
- an inflamed throat often displaying white spots
- a fever
- a headache
- an earache
- enlarged and tender neck lymph nodes
- snoring
- sleep apnoea
- unpleasant smelling breath (halitosis).

Occasionally, tonsillitis can cause temporary deafness or quinsy (an abscess around the tonsils). Complications from streptococcal tonsillitis include;
- Pneumonia (infection causing an inflammation of the lungs)
- Nephritis (inflammation of one or both kidneys)
- Osteomyelitis (infection of bone and bone marrow)
- Rheumatic fever (an autoimmune disorder).

Treatment of tonsillitis

There are several ways of treating the onset of tonsillitis and these include;
- bed rest
- drink plenty of fluids
- analgesic drug (painkiller) e.g. paracetemol
- antibiotic drugs.

145

If there are recurring bouts of severe tonsillitis, the tonsils may be surgically removed (Tonsillectomy). This operation can also be carried out if quinsy is present. This procedure is also carried out on diphtheria (an acute bacterial illness) carriers because the tonsils may 'seed' the infection.

If necessary the adenoids can be removed at the same time, this operation is known as a T&A.

Adenoidal conditions

Because the lymph nodes called adenoids usually shrink after the age of five and disappear altogether by puberty, conditions are normally restricted to this age group. If there have been repeated childhood respiratory tract infections adenoid hypertrophy (enlargement) may occur. The passage from the nose to the throat can be obstructed and this will cause;
- breathing through the mouth
- a 'nasally' voice
- snoring and possible sleep apnoea
- a possibly blocked Eustachian tube, causing middle ear infection (Otitis media) and impaired hearing.

Treatment of adenoidal conditions

A doctor will inspect the back of the throat using a mirror with a light attached, sometimes an X-ray will be taken. The infection is usually treated with antibiotic drugs but sometimes the infections will recur. Recurrence in children or in those adults with recurring sore throats, ear pain, hearing dysfunction or who snore because of hypertrophied adenoid or tonsil tissue will be treated surgically.

The surgery can either be the removal of adenoid material (adenoidectomy) or a T&A (adenotonsillectomy) which also removes tonsil tissue.

Cancer of the larynx (voice box)

Causes

Although the causes of this type of malignant cancer, which represents 2% of all cancers, is not known it is most common in heavy smokers, is associated with high alcohol consumption and affects people over 60 especially men.

Symptoms

Hoarseness is the main symptom, especially when the tumour originates on the vocal cords. Elsewhere, it will be unnoticed until it is in the advanced stages when there will be difficulty in breathing and swallowing, throat discomfort and coughing up blood.

Diagnosis

The larynx will be examined (laryngoscopy) either directly with a mirror or indirectly with a viewing instrument to see if there is a tumour. A biopsy will be done in a hospital under local or general anaesthetic to determine whether the growth is benign or malignant and if the larynx shows signs of early cancerous growth.

Treatment

Early discovery of a tumour is important, if the tumour is small the outcome is favourable; a small cancer of the vocal cords, which is treated with radiotherapy or laser, has a 95% chance of cure.

For a large or unresponsive tumour, partial or total removal of the larynx (laryngectomy) is considered unless the patient is elderly or weak. If a laryngectomy is carried out the patient must master new techniques with the aid of a speech therapist for producing speech through the stoma (opening) in the neck. There are different devices available to help generate speech. The cure rate varies according to site and extent of the tumour.

If the tumour has spread through the larynx or to other parts of the throat, and possibly the body, treatment is with radiotherapy and anticancer drugs, symptoms are usually relieved and temporarily the spread of the disease is halted.

The National Association of Laryngectomee Clubs (NALC) can be a useful reference point for patients who have had, or are considering a laryngectomy.

CHAPTER 9: COMPLEMENTARY AND OTHER THERAPIES

Introduction

Complementary Therapies and Disciplines supplemental to General Medicine

Complementary therapies and disciplines supplemental to general medicine, such as osteopathy and chiropractic, have had an increasingly important role to play in helping and treating many conditions. Their availability gives people another treatment option and generally the wait to consult a complementary therapist is much less than seeing a medical specialist. Because of the scope of this book and the veritable explosion of therapies and their scope especially in the last ten years I have regrettably had to omit some of the therapies which are available and which can help with medical, including ENT, conditions.

I should repeat that I hold the view that the concept is of complementary therapy and not alternative therapy and that if someone has an acute or chronic disease or physical pain attention should be sought from a medical practitioner. The medical practitioner should have access to a patient's records and to the necessary testing and diagnostic equipment, which are essential to diagnose certain conditions prior to their treatment.

The main aim of all therapists should be to treat both the condition; its cause and symptoms together with any other underlying problems - physical, emotional or spiritual or a combination of these - this is the holistic approach. Obviously, there may be time and economic constraints involved. Time constraints should be less in the complementary therapy scenario where treatment sessions are able, on the whole, to last longer than in most medical practices or hospitals. Normally, complementary therapy has to be paid for by the patient but increasingly costs are being reimbursed by private medical insurance companies and some treatments are now available free on the National Health Service to which the individual normally makes financial contribution. If a person adopts the private healthcare route regular financial costs have to be made.

It is important that both parties assume their responsibilities and the patient/client should understand and be informed (politely) that he/she has an important part to play in the healing process. It is for this reason that advice given by the therapist at the end of a session could range from a series of stretches and weight bearing exercises to be carried out to a series of affirmations which should be repeated each day depending on the condition being treated. Not only should this advice help the restorative process but it should also play a significant part, hopefully, in preventing a recurrence of the problem/condition.

Choosing a therapist

It is important for someone who wishes to be treated by a therapist outside the framework of the National Health Service (NHS) to try and check if he/she is properly qualified, accountable and an ethical professional. Some therapists such as most chiropractors and osteopaths belong to their main regulating body (some excellent chiropractors and osteopaths do not however). Other therapists do not belong to regulating bodies but belong to reputable organisations with codes of practice and ethical guidelines.

The best recommendation in health care, as in most other service industries, is recommendation from a family member, friend, colleague or GP practice. Many therapists do advertise in telephone directories, newspapers and magazines or in public places but this can be impersonal in the first instance and if the therapist asks questions over the telephone or on the internet this can cause the client/patient some embarrassment and possible confusion.

Costs will vary between therapies and therapists due to the complexity of treatment, geographical location, experience and skill of the therapist.

Having chosen a therapist the client/patient could ask the following questions;
- are you competent to treat my condition?
- how will you be treating my condition?
- are you insured to carry out the proposed treatment?
- are you a member of a recognised professional organisation?
- how long will the treatments take, what is the cost and how many will I have to have?
- have you much success in treating my condition?
- will I have to do anything to help speed my recovery?
- will you be in contact with my GP about my treatment?

The client/patient should expect the following;
- to be treated in a professional, safe and courteous manner
- the therapist and treatment area should be clean and safe
- the treatment and its implications to be fully explained
- a case study/consultation form to be completed prior to commencement of the first treatment
- a timescale of treatments and advice to be offered for some self help action to be done by the client/patient.

The case study/medical history

The case study will include questions such as;
- current and past state of health (physical/emotional/spiritual) including current symptoms and pain and sleep patterns
- medication currently being taken
- any other practitioner being/been seen

149

- family details in case of heredity factor
- diet and exercise
- work and leisure activities.

The information in the following section is only a guideline and a qualified therapist/practitioner will be able to treat the individual correctly on a personal basis using information supplied by the client/patient and his/her own skill and experience. It is important not to self diagnose; self treating should be done after consulting a therapist/practitioner.

The treatments covered are;
- **Acupuncture and Auricular Therapy**
- **Alexander Technique**
- **Aromatherapy**
- **Ayurvedic Medicine**
- **Biofeedback**
- **Chiropractic and McTimoney Chiropractic**
- **Chinese Herbalism**
- **Western Herbalism**
- **Homeopathy**
- **Hypnotherapy**
- **Kinesiology and Health Kinesiology**
- **Massage**
- **Naturopathy**
- **Osteopathy and Cranial Osteopathy**
- **Cranio-Sacral Therapy**
- **Reflexology**
- **Shiatsu and Acupressure.**

Acupuncture and Auricular Therapy

Acupuncture

This treatment which originated in China has been used for over 5,000 years. Very fine needles are used to stimulate specific points to balance the movement of 'Chi' energy along meridian lines. Meridian points which relate to ear and sinus problems are the liver, spleen, kidney, triple heater and small intestine. These meridians will be concentrated on but other meridians will also be treated. Other techniques which are available include moxibustion, cupping, electro acupuncture and herbs.

Many ENT conditions can be treated including neuralgia and tinnitus.

Selected Auricular Therapy
Stimulation Points of The Ear

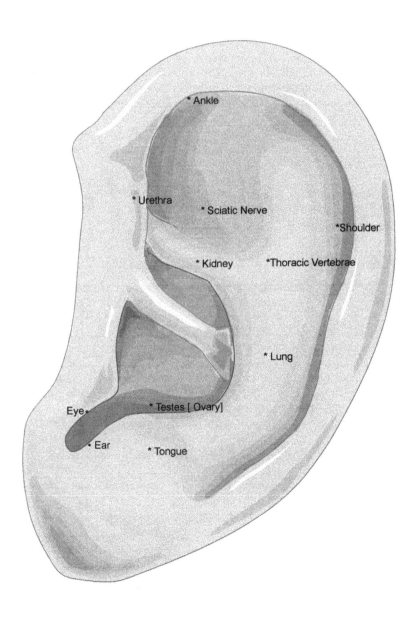

Auricular Therapy

Auricular means external ear and auricular therapy concentrates on over 300 acupressure points on the auricle. Again this therapy originated thousands of years ago in China but it had a renaissance when Dr Paul Nogier a French acupuncturist revived and updated it in the 1960s. The shape of the ear resembles either a foetus in the womb or a kidney and the points on the ear relate to specific areas or organs of the body.

By stimulating the points with needles, magnets, ball bearings or seeds the corresponding area of the body is stimulated; sometimes these items are taped to the ear for a week and the patient can press on them to extend the treatment. As well as stimulating points relating to the ear, nose throat and sinuses the whole auricle is stimulated during a treatment.

This treatment is less invasive than acupuncture and is less traumatic for those nervous of needles.

Auricular therapy will bring temporary relief from neuralgia but body acupuncture should be more effective. It should also help ear infections, sinus problems and tinnitus.

Alexander Technique

The Alexander Technique is named after its inventor, Frederick Matthias Alexander, an Australian actor who at the turn of the 20th century realised that the relationship of the head and neck related to the rest of the body and so also to correct body use. This was described as 'The Primary Control' theory. He thought that when the head, neck and back work harmoniously this was a key factor in the balance of the whole person - body and mind. When harmony is restored to the whole body specific problems disappear. While good posture is also a key to good health, the Alexander Technique, which is taught to a pupil by a teacher in a 1 to 1 situation, aims to get people to move with ease and grace and with increased balance and poise.

Alexander also thought that we have become more interested in mental tasks rather than physical ones and that our occupations have restricted our natural movements which have become more repetitive which have led from childhood to aches and pains. All our movements should be considered instead of being automatic/inhibited as this will lead to them being carried out correctly. It is important to practice the correct movements (the Technique) repetitively to gain maximum benefit.

There should be a course of about thirty lessons, although the number will depend on the pupil's needs. During the lessons the teacher may;

- ask why the pupil has come and what is hoped to be achieved
- identify and unravel the pupil's patterns of unconscious misuse and restore natural reflexes
- ask the pupil to carry out movements and explain how they can be done correctly and effortlessly
- encourage the pupil to let go of spinal tension with postural work on a massage table in the semi-supine position
- give the pupil homework which may include lying in the semi-supine position daily so as to lengthen and relax the spine.

While many people generally improve stress related conditions the main ENT conditions which can be helped are fatigue, rhinitis, tonsillitis, sinusitis, breathing problems, eye strain, headaches and migraines and neck problems.

Aromatherapy

The history of using aromatic oils as a healing tool goes back many thousands of years; indeed the Egyptian physician Imhotep who became a god of healing recommended their use over 6,000 years ago. Both ancient Athens and medieval London got rid of the plague by using aromatic fumigations and essential oils. The modern father of aromatherapy was Rene-Maurice Gattefosse, a French chemist, who in the 1930s after burning his hand in the laboratory plunged his hand into a vat of lavender oil and amazingly his recovery was quick without infection and no scarring. Other French pioneers, including Madame Marguerite Maury who first used essential oils in massage,developed further this therapy which aims to heal the mind and body and restore balance to the overall system.

The most effective therapeutic use of oils is through massaging the skin, although they can be used in steam inhalations, baths, compresses, diffusers and vaporisers. There are about 150 essential oils which are aromatic essences extracted from various parts of plants, grasses and trees. Each of them have a unique scent and healing properties; all of them are antiseptics, some are stimulating, relaxing, pain relieving, antidepressant, diuretic, aid digestion and so on.

Oils are extracted using different processes and their cost reflects the amount of raw material and its purity needed in the process. Synthetic substitutes do not give the same results. Each oil has over 100 chemical constituents and it is these which when working together enable physical and emotional healing to be facilitated. The scent of the oils reaches the limbic part of the brain via the olfactory nervous system and the result is that memories are triggered and our moods and emotions are altered.

It is important to remember that when essential oils (excepting lavender oil) are used in massage they are not applied neat directly on the skin but are mixed/blended beforehand with a carrier oil such as almond oil or grape seed oil. If they are used neat there is a great danger that they will burn the skin.

Unless under strict medical supervision, essential oils must not be ingested; they must also be kept away from the eyes. If oils are drunk, especially by children they should eat plenty of bread and drink milk with a doctor being consulted. If oils are splashed on the skin or in the eyes they should be flushed off with water.

Aromatherapy massage oils are soon absorbed into the body and they work on the skin almost immediately. A warm environment and warm therapist hands will speed the absorption rate. The oils exit the body up to fourteen hours later.

It would be prudent to consult a qualified aromatherapist before using essential oils at home. Some oils have however been used safely and these include lavender, tea tree, eucalyptus or Olbas.

Before having a treatment an aromatherapist will;
● ask why you have come and take a full case study
● decide which oils will be best and which to avoid using - pregnancy, sensitive skin, abnormal blood pressure and epilepsy are contraindications against the use of certain oils
● ask about stress levels, emotions and moods
● ask if there any oils which are preferred by the client.

During the treatment session which is normally carried out on a massage couch the therapist will use the most appropriate blend of oils and use mainly gentle Swedish massage strokes with some shiatsu techniques being incorporated. A treatment will normally last for up to one hour. The first session incorporating the consultation will take longer - this is normal practice for all therapies. It is often better to leave the oils on the body for a few hours so that they can be absorbed fully and the aroma will be remembered longer; if possible do not wear expensive clothes to a treatment.

At the conclusion of the treatment the aromatherapist will explain possible reactions which may be experienced and oils may be given to the client to use at home possibly in the bath.

Many ENT problems such as; ear infections, tinnitus, tonsillitis, laryngitis, sinus problems, rhinitis, headaches, excessive ear wax, loss of smell, colds and flu can be treated with aromatherapy.

Ayurvedic Medicine

Ayurvedic medicine is over 3,000 years old and originated in India. It is part of an overall philosophy called Veda which is the knowledge of how the world works. Ayurveda is Sanskrit for 'meaning of life' and combines science and philosophy which gives the answers for attaining holistic health. Its many components - detoxification, diet, exercise, herbs and mental and emotional strengthening exercises combine together to give a way of life not an occasional treatment.

The fundamental concept in Ayurveda is that everything is composed of energy ('prana') and that we are constantly changing in positive or negative ways. To achieve maximum positive changes life must be lived in balance. As everyone is different so the balance of energies which is good for one person may lead to ill health in someone else.

A good constitution is the best way of defending against illness. Ayurveda will try to work with your body rather than changing it. There are three vital energies ('doshas' - a Sanskrit word) in the body; vatha, pitha and kapha which govern our constitution so we can we can be described as a pitha type, kapha type, pitha/kapha type etc. Each dosha determines illness, constitution, hair colour, type of food which should be eaten and every part of life. Good health happens when all three doshas are in harmony.

Ayurveda practitioners also have to take into consideration the five elements and five senses - ether/sound, air/touch, fire/sight, water/taste and earth/smell. Good digestion is considered the key to good health. Emotions can produce toxins which can manifest as bloating and intestinal pain.

A practitioner will;
● ask detailed questions about health
● study the way you move
● check the fingers and thumbs as they relate to the organs and elements
● take the pulse in three points.

Treatment will vary and it can include detoxification using different methods, yoga, exercise and herbal remedies. Conventional medicines must be continued. Ayurveda is effective for many ENT conditions such as colds and flu, sinusitis, rhinitis and tonsillitis.

Biofeedback

Biofeedback is a method of relaxing when the body is attached by electrodes to machinery which measures the body's (temperature, pulse, respiration and blood pressure) and brain's reaction to stress; control of these elements when stressed is learnt. Physiological changes are registered on a screen and eventually you recognise the effects of relaxation without machinery. Biofeedback is one of many methods of relaxing including visualization, tense/release relaxation, passive relaxation and applied relaxation.

Chiropractic and McTimoney Chiropractic

Chiropractic
Manipulation of bones goes back many centuries to the ancient Chinese and Greeks but it was not until 1895 that the Canadian magnetic healer Daniel David Palmer founded chiropractic.

154

Chiropractic works on the body's musculo-skeletal system especially the spine and through specific examination and manipulation chiropractors can treat the many conditions associated with the system. Chiropractors do not deal exclusively with spinal problems but they can treat headaches, ankle pain and ear pain caused by misalignment of the ear's ossicle bones.

While chiropractic is similar in theory and philosophy to osteopathy it differs in different ways;

- chiropractors concentrate on one joint at a time; osteopaths can stretch several joints at one time
- chiropractors use x-rays more than osteopaths
- spinal manipulation is fundamental to chiropractors; it is not central to osteopaths.

Chiropractors diagnose using palpation, observation and x-rays. Manipulation of joints takes the joint further than the normal range of movement and this is achieved by using any or some of over 100 techniques. The most common of these are;

- direct thrust techniques - rapid, forceful movements which are often accompanied by cracking noise when the gas bubbles in fluid burst
- indirect thrust techniques - more gentle movements than direct thrusts; the joint is gently stretched for a few minutes over a towel, pad or wedge
- soft tissue techniques - relax joints prior to adjustments and often used to release 'trigger points' which are similar to reflex points.

A chiropractor will;

- take a detailed case study
- examine the patient, especially the spine
- ask the patient to move, bend, walk etc
- carry out routine medical tests - take pulse, check blood pressure and reflexes
- static palpation of the joints
- take x-rays to help decide which techniques to use or if a treatment should be carried out (tumours and fractures would obviate treatment)
- conduct treatment and give after advice about posture, diet and lifting.

Reactions to this treatment, like all other treatments, can vary from being relaxed to being energised. It is also possible that the patient may be sore for a few days.

Chiropractic will help all the ENT conditions listed under the section on osteopathy. Middle ear infections including 'Glue Ear' are helped by chiropractic adjustments of the neck and upper back which restore proper joint motion and so the Eustachian tube should drain properly with the body's immune system able to fight infection.

McTimoney Chiropractic

John McTimoney (1914- 1980) was treated successfully with chiropractic for an arm injury and was enthused to train in the profession. He expanded the basic philosophy by taking into account joints in the arms and hands, legs and feet, thorax and skull as well as the spine and pelvis. Practitioners take a full case study and check the spine and angle of the pelvis. Misalignment of the pelvis gives the impression that one leg is longer than the other.

McTimoney chiropractic is gentle using manipulation by the hands only and a practitioner looks at the whole body rather than just the spine.

Cranio- Sacral therapy

Cranio -sacral therapy is derived from cranial osteopathy. It is similar in technique and philosophy but does not have the same detailed examination of patients. A cranial osteopath will have had full osteopathic training and most likely be a member of the General Council and Register of Osteopaths. A cranio-sacral therapist may have a background of osteopathy or not.

Chinese Herbalism

Chinese herbalism is part of traditional Chinese Medicine (TCM) which is over 5,000 year old and is becoming increasingly popular in the West. While Western scientists extract the active ingredients to suppress symptoms of a condition the Chinese use herbs to treat the person not their disease. The herbs are seen as preventative as well as curative for mind, body and spiritual problems. Herbs can be used either in conjunction with acupuncture or on their own often when the body is too weak to have much energy or if someone does not want needles.

All TCM works on balancing the body and this balance is brought about understanding and working on concepts of yin and yang; Chi energy which likes blood and moisture flows around the body along the various meridians; the five elements (metal, water, wood, fire and earth) and eight principles.

A Chinese herbalist will examine using four procedures;
* looking - general appearance, state of eyes and tongue, colour of face
* listening and smelling - breathing patterns, speech and cough
* asking - questions about you, lifestyle, medical history, symptoms; similar questions that other types of therapist will ask
* touching - palpating the part of the body where there is pain or a rash and taking three pulses in each wrist which will give twenty different pulse qualities.

The herbal prescription is designed to balance body and mind and may be dispensed after the first treatment or a week later after a mini check up.

Chinese herbalism is good for many ENT conditions including; ear infections including glue ear, tonsillitis, laryngitis, sinusitis, allergic rhinitis, travel sickness, headaches, migraines, colds and flu.

Western Herbalism

Herbalism has been practised in the West for many centuries and material such as willow bark and digitalis from the foxglove which produce aspirin and dixogin (for heart problems) respectively are probably known to most people. Herbs contain many active healing chemical constituents and compounds including vitamins, minerals and volatile oils. The aims of using herbs include fighting infection, reducing inflammation and improving circulation and their whole is stronger than their parts.

Correctly used after prescription by a qualified herbalist they should work effectively without side effects. They are designed to support body systems rather than symptoms. The main philosophical difference between Chinese and Western herbalism is that the Chinese tradition is the importance of understanding yin and yang and the flow of Chi around the body. Two of the main practical differences are that a Chinese herbalist will rely more on smelling and detailed pulse taking.

The Western herbalist will;
- take a full case study and ask about your personality and stress levels
- ask about childhood, job and leisure pursuits
- ask about how you feel about your different bodily systems
- ask about the home and work environments
- if qualified, carry out a physical examination e.g. take pulse and blood pressure and test reflexes
- assess how a condition was started
- prescribe a suitable treatment and offer advice on diet, exercise and relaxation
- refer you to another practitioner where necessary - doctor, osteopath or chiropractor
- ask you to return for a second treatment and advise that the remedies may make you feel worse before feeling better.

The herbal treatments include;

- **tinctures**
- **infusions**
- **decoctions**
- **tablets and capsules**
- **creams and ointments**
- **hot or cold compresses**
- **poultices**
- **suppositories and douches**
- **herbal baths**
- **fresh herbs to be incorporated into the diet**

Western herbalism is effective for many ENT conditions especially, sinusitis, tonsillitis, laryngitis, allergic rhinitis, travel sickness, headaches, migraines, infections including glue ear, eyestrain, colds and flu.

Homeopathy

Homeopathy which treats the body as a whole and helps it to heal itself is a holistic therapy which has as its cornerstone the philosophy of 'treating like with like'. Its origins date back to Hippocrates in Greece in the 5th century BC when his understanding of disease and how it affects us rather than its remedies made him homeopathic in outlook. Homeopathy was lost until it was rediscovered by the German physician and chemist Samuel Hahnemann (1755 - 1843). Hahnemann was outraged by the poor hygiene and savage, often dangerous, medical treatments of that time. After reading a book by Dr William Cullen he devised a theory that the severity of symptoms and the healing responses depended on the individual, he also constructed a symptoms picture of each patient before deciding which remedy to prescribe -these pictures are still valid today.

Homeopathy uses a substance that while causing symptoms of illness in a well person can also cure similar symptoms when they are in a state of illness. This idea is the opposite of conventional medicine which treats illness with an antidote rather than with a similar substance. A homeopath will treat someone suffering from a headache with a minute amount of something which may cause a headache if given in a large amount rather than paracetemol which may cure a headache if prescribed by a conventional doctor. There are in excess of 2,000 homeopathic remedies and they should match the patient's condition. As well as homeopathic remedies, tissue salts can be prescribed.

Tissue salts are prepared from mineral sources and homeopathic remedies are made from animal, vegetable and mineral extracts. The remedy is diluted to such an extent that there is no risk of any side effects. The dilution can be as much as 1:1,000. The dilution is finally made into tablets, pills or powder.

Homeopaths think that symptoms of a condition are an expression of the body fighting back to heal itself and these symptoms should be supported and not repressed as would be the case with conventional medicine. Remedies are prescribed following Hahnemann's three principles;

● the law of similars - an introduced artificial disease will push out an original one without causing long term suffering because it is temporary
● the minimum dose - extreme dilution enhance curative properties of a substance
● whole person prescribing - prescription after studying the whole person.

Homeopaths think their remedies contain an energy which is the curing agent that activates our own internal healing power similar to 'ki', 'chi' or 'prana'. This concept is difficult to grasp and so far impossible to prove but with the millions of people who swear by homeopathy there must be something to it.

Homeopaths also believe that treatment works following the **three Laws of Cure**;

1.   **the remedy works from the top of the body downwards**
2.   **the remedy works from inwards to outwards and from major to minor organs**
3.   **the symptoms clear in order of appearance and that emotional problems clear before physical ones.**

Homeopaths also examine constitutional types; an individual has inherited as well as acquired physical, mental and emotional characteristics and that the remedy can be matched to these to improve health.

A homeopath will;

● take a full case study and ask many questions about your background
● ask about past illnesses and family health
● ask if you are up to changes in your life
● types of food you like and whether you react to hot and cold
● prescribe a remedy which can be altered at following sessions.

While some people get better quickly, for others it takes longer and some people are not cured at all - this situation is the same for all therapies. While homeopathy can help with any condition, in the field of ENT conditions it is well suited for; tonsillitis, laryngitis, ear infections, tinnitus, sinusitis, headaches, migraines, eye strain, colds and flu and travel sickness.

Hypnotherapy

Hypnotherapy is a type of psychotherapy that induces patients to enter a state of trance, between waking and sleeping, so that healing or change can happen. The father of hypnosis was Franz Anton Mesmer (1734 -1815) who was born near Lake Constance and who worked in Austria and France. Although there is the stage entertainment side of hypnosis, it is effective for pain relief by enabling the mind to accept pain reducing information which is what the subject wants to hear. Hypnosis also facilitates the rejection of beliefs and patterns of behaviour and thereby can be useful for overcoming fears and phobias. It is important for the subject to want to cooperate with the hypnotist to bring about a change.

Hypnotists think, like other therapists, that the mind and body are linked and that emotional problems can be the cause of physical illness and that an injured or amputated limb can cause depression or other emotional ill. The mind's subconscious has the ability to activate the body's physical healing mechanism.

It is thought that the mind functions on two levels; the conscious and the subconscious. The subconscious rules the conscious in desires and all mental and physical functions - from regulating heart rate to memory storage. The subconscious is the real you and the source of human energy. Without using the subconscious it will not be possible to fulfil one's full potential. Because the subconscious will believe anything it is told when the subject is in a trance the hypnotist can suggest positive thoughts to replace negative ones such as giving up drinking alcohol.

During a treatment session the hypnotist will;
- ask why the subject has come, explain what hypnotism is (and isn't) and reassure the subject that the therapy is safe and that the subject will not do anything he/she does not want to do
- build up a relationship with the subject based on trust
- explain that common problems such as smoking or being overweight may need less treatment sessions than long term physical or deep seated emotional conditions
- relax the subject and use appropriate hypnosis techniques (hypnosis might not be done during the first appointment) in either a chair or on a couch
- at the end of a session bring the subject back to a conscious state
- possibly teach the subject self hypnosis techniques for use between treatments.

Hypnotherapy can be used for many physical, mental and psychosomatic problems. It is often associated with helping habit and addiction problems and also conditions related to a person's history and their stress levels. Many ENT conditions can be treated including neuralgia, eyestrain, headaches, migraines and tinnitus which can be triggered by different causes including high stress levels.

Kinesiology and Health Kinesiology

Kinesiology
Kinesiology is a diagnostic therapy which analyses the cause of illness or disease rather than diagnosing a specific condition. It was originally systemised by Henry and Florence Kendall in 1949 who wrote a book called 'Muscle testing and function'. This book was in response to work carried out by R W Lovett, an orthopaedic surgeon, who in the 1920s developed a test for grading the strength of muscles. An American chiropractor Dr George J Goodheart, then furthered this work in the 1960s and he developed a system of massaging certain points to correct muscle weakness. Goodheart also realised that the muscle response was affected by the meridians as used by Acupuncturists and Shiatsu practitioners. As these meridians are thought to be part of the energy system of our body Goodheart recognised that if there was an imbalance in the meridian it would have an effect on the response of the muscle when tested.

A kinesiologist will;
- take a detailed case study before the start of the first treatment session
- ask about your work and lifestyle
- ask if you wish to proceed as it is necessary to want the treatment to work
- test the muscle by asking you to resist against a pressing down on an arm or leg - good resistance is a sign of health in the related organ, weakening indicates an energy imbalance in the related organ
- test for food intolerance by placing a test vial of food on the jaw or navel
- carry out the treatment possibly utilising other therapies in which he/she may be qualified.

Kinesiology aims to find and correct small problems before they become serious   especially food sensitivities, aches, stiff joints and digestive problems. Neuralgia, ear infections including glue ear, tinnitus, tonsillitis, laryngitis and headaches are some of the ENT problems which can be treated.

Health Kinesiology

Health Kinesiology was developed from Goodheart's Kinesiology in the 1970s by Dr Jimmy Scott, a psychologist and while its basic structure was formed by 1981 it is still evolving up to this time. When Dr Scott initially saw kinesiology being demonstrated, he was as most people are at that time and still now, both fascinated and highly sceptical.

Health Kinesiology has been successfully used for both humans and animals, although in the UK it is not to be used professionally without the consent of a vet. A client does not need to understand why he/she has a problem, as Health Kinesiology helps the physical body function more efficiently and enables the client to feel fulfilled and happier. People do not have to be physically ill to consult a Health Kinesiologist although most people do come due to some disease in their life i.e. emotional problems, poor performance at school, no diagnosis from the GP but the problem still exists; lack of esteem, amongst many others.

When a client visits a Health Kinesiologist he/she will take a comprehensive health history which will give an insight into the individual problems of each person. Perhaps a client's ear problems stem from sinusitis or catarrh, or it may be that the client has a weakened immune system, which then leads to the ear problems.

By using muscle testing a Health Kinesiologist will check for imbalances in the client's energy system. This will be shown by a client giving a weakened muscle response when a muscle is taken through a range of movements. Each treatment is individually tailored to the client by muscle testing and using a menu of corrections. Some of the corrections may work on clearing allergies or intolerance, along with a variety of corrections to improve the energy system. Many people are not aware that the symptoms that they suffer from could be a reaction to something to which they have intolerance. When stressed a body will show more symptoms of allergies and intolerance, this is why it is so hard to pinpoint the actual cause. Excess of mucous in some people can be caused by intolerance to dairy products and when finding a weakened muscle response a Health Kinesiologist can use a specific correction to help. This correction is called a SET technique, which will help a client detoxify and enable the client to deal with the substance more effectively.

Within the Health Kinesiology menu of corrections, magnets may be placed on the body while holding acupressure points. With ear problems the magnet may be placed on the sinus area or even the throat. The throat area is where the chakra is which relates to the ears and throat. Chakras are energy centres at certain places through-out the body and these chakras can relate to the health of nearby organs and glands. If this chakra energy is out of balance, perhaps due to an emotional problem or an injury, then the related areas can become out of balance too.

At each treatment a Health Kinesiologist works up a set of corrections, which are totally individual to that particular client, therefore no two treatments are ever the same, as no two people are the same. Generally in most other treatments of ear problems a similar route is followed, however with Health Kinesiology no set pattern fits as this therapy looks at us as the individuals we are.

Massage

Massage is one of the oldest therapies in the world, probably predating acupuncture, and was popular with the Greeks and Romans. The act of touching and stroking the body is one of the most natural in the world. Its healing benefits were recognised by the Catholic Church up to the middle ages but at that point it fell into disuse. The father of therapeutic massage was Professor Per Henrik Ling (1776 - 1839) a Swedish gymnast turned masseur who codified moves and theory into Swedish massage which is still being taught and practised worldwide to this day.

Massage is the manipulation of the body's soft tissues using a number of different strokes depending on the purpose of the massage. Normally, the therapist will only use hands but the feet, elbows and forearms can also be utilised. As well as improving bodily function by reducing muscle tension, emotional release can also be gained especially by a holistic therapist.
Massage is the basis of other therapies such as aromatherapy, shiatsu, physiotherapy (in the UK, the foundation of an organisation which was later to become the Chartered Society of Physiotherapists was laid at a meeting of the Society of Trained Masseuses in the Strand, London in December 1894 who wanted to be acknowledged for their professionalism and ethical approach), Chinese and Ayurvedic medicine.

Massage can either be relaxing or stimulating depending on its purpose. There are many moves including gliding, stroking, kneading, hacking, tapping, vibrating, frictioning, knuckling and wringing. Massage sessions can last from ten minutes to two hours although the average is one hour and oils or creams can be used. Massage can be done with the person lightly clothed, wearing underwear or naked. Modesty is always a priority and towels are draped over the body except for the area being worked on. It is better to work on a massage couch with a face hole or head extension; on a mat on the floor or with an ergonomic massage chair rather than on a bed which gives under pressure. Electric massagers can also be used.

The Golden rule of massage

Although massage comes in many forms - stress relief, sports massage, Indian Head Massage, Swedish massage, remedial massage its action can all be summed up in the author's mantra about massage;

- widening (of the body)
- lengthening (of the body)
- deepening (of the body)
- pressure
- timing.

A massage therapist will;

- take a case history
- ask about the current state of health
- ask what medication is currently being taken

- ask whether any alcohol or a heavy meal has been consumed just prior to the treatment
- explain how the massage will be conducted and what oils or creams are going to be used
- check for contraindications against a massage such as broken bones or an infectious skin complaint
- check that the correct massage pressure is being used and that the client is comfortable
- leave the client alone for a few minutes at the cessation of the treatment so that he/she can recover from being 'spaced out' by the treatment
- recommend that the client drink some water at the end of the session to help with the elimination of toxins
- give some post treatment advice such as diet and lifestyle changes which could be made.

Like all other therapies the effect of the treatment is unpredictable. Some people may get better quickly; others may feel worse before they get better. The therapist should advise the client beforehand about this.

Massage of the neck and face is very good for treating the cause of some headaches and migraines such as eyestrain or stiff necks; tonsillitis, stimulating blood and lymphatic circulation in the head area, ear infections, sinus drainage and helping with TMJ dysfunction.

Naturopathy

Naturopathy, like many other therapies can be associated with Hippocrates who is considered to be the father of medicine and whose oath all medical doctors should abide by. His adoption of diet, fasting, hydrotherapy, exercise and manipulative techniques is used today as an alternative to drug treatment. Naturopathy has been increasingly used since the 1970s especially in the USA and is a system where natural resources help the body heal itself. It is based on three principles;
1.   the vital force - the body has its own curative force which fights illness
2.   disease is a natural state when the whole body is not working properly
3.   the symptoms of disease are evidence that the body is trying to heal itself and that the vital force is trying to balance the body.

Naturopaths think that treatment should be holistic and natural, good posture and nutrition is relevant and that the Law of Cure applies (see also the section about homeopathy). Diagnosis can depend on utilisation of a number of different methods;

- medical testing such as blood pressure and pulse taking
- observation and palpation (if the naturopath is an osteopath)
- Biotypography which classifies people by their shape i.e. endomorphs: soft and round, ectomorphs: long and lean and mesomorphs: muscular and stocky. Each shape type is prone to different illnesses
- iridology - iris of the eye diagnosis
- mineral analysis - hair and sweat can be tested for minerals and trace elements
- Bioelectric dowsing which takes readings from saliva, blood, nail clippings or hair.

Treatment depends on the training and qualifications of the naturopath and can include;
- diet
- fasting
- hydrotherapy
- osteopathy
- psychotherapy
- colonic irrigation.

The naturopath will;
- take a case study
- enquire about diet and bowel movements
- ask about relationships with others
- ask about sleep patterns
- ask about the work and leisure situation
- carry out medical tasks
- recommend a treatment regime which may include diet, a detox fast and exercise - in essence a change in lifestyle.

Naturopathy can treat many ENT conditions including; ear infections including glue ear, tonsillitis, laryngitis, neuralgia, allergic rhinitis, sinusitis, colds and flu and headaches and migraine.

Osteopathy and Cranial Osteopathy

Osteopathy

Osteopathy is becoming increasingly popular and accepted as a treatment and in the UK over five million people visit a practitioner; in the USA more that 100 million visits are made. It is a system devised in 1874 by an American doctor Andrew Taylor Still who was also an engineer. He studied body mechanics and postulated that 'structure governs function' and that muscle tension and misaligned bones place unnecessary strain on the whole body. The causes of the strain can be physical injury, poor posture, and emotional problems including anger, anxiety and fear. If the body, especially the spine which protects the spinal cord and the central nervous system, can be adjusted the strain would be relieved and the body would work better and heal itself. Osteopathy was introduced into the UK by Jon Martin Littlejohn in 1917 who had studied at the Kirksville School of osteopathy, Missouri which Andrew Taylor Still had founded.

Osteopathy is a manipulative therapy which works on the body's structure to restore health by relieving pain and improving mobility. All parts of the body and mind are interrelated so it is possible for internal problems such as a malfunctioning kidney to lead to lower back pain. With manipulation it is possible to restore overall health, osteopaths also concentrate on easing muscular tension as muscles use up a great deal of energy when they contract. Tense muscles are more prone to damage and they impede the flow of blood and lymph which are the supply and waste systems of the body. Manipulation also has a positive effect on the working of the nervous system and related glands and hormones.

Osteopaths use many techniques, which they consider as tools, depending on the muscles to be treated;

- soft tissue manipulation - on skin, connective tissue and muscles
- articulatory techniques (including traction) - stretch muscles or ligaments
- high, medium or low velocity thrust - this is used mainly on the spine. Cracking or popping noises are merely joints releasing themselves
- muscle energy techniques - used on tight muscles, especially caused by sports injuries
- indirect techniques - very gentle mainly to reduce stress; cranial osteopathy uses these techniques.

An osteopath;

- will take a case study
- assess body framework and posture
- check the spine, hips, pelvis, legs, chest and muscle tone
- ask you to stand, move and lean forward, backward and to the side
- may use x-rays
- will give after care advice including diet, lifestyle and exercise advice.

In a very few cases it is possible that joint manipulation may leave the client feeling sore for a few days after the treatment. Neck problems, hay fever, ear infections including glue ear, dizziness, headaches, migraines, sinusitis, tinnitus and TMJ jaw dysfunction are some of the ENT problems which can be helped by osteopathy.

Osteopathy can be very successful in treating 'glue ear'; if it is treated manually there is a 75-80% success rate and if dietary change is incorporated this rises to 90-95%. Over 40% of children and adults have a problem digesting dairy produce and this is linked to an over-production of mucus. Osteopaths take into consideration mechanical and structural dysfunction as well as congestive dysfunction and allergies. Mechanical can be due to a traumatic birth process i.e. forceps or suction, caesarean, prolonged labour etc. Congestion, whether dietary or viral, is caused by mucus membrane irritation to the goblet cells which secrete mucus within the epithelium.

When osteopaths treat children it is vital that the parents are fully committed. Osteopathy is cost effective for parents and the NHS regarding the cost of drug and speech therapy and operative care. Manually it is less traumatic because;

- no general anaesthetic is needed
- the adenoids and palatine tonsils do not have to be removed
- the tympanic membrane is not scarred by the insertion of a grommet (myringotomy).

There is no chance for post operative infection as may be the case with the insertion of grommets and possible reinsertion of grommets with consequent scarring is not an option.
Dr Tony Matthews, DO has treated 300 patients since 1992 with a success rate of 90-95% and his treatment protocol can be taught to parents with learning reinforced by a full colour video showing the complete ear and sinus treatment together with instruction sheets about palpation. It is essential that a suitably qualified practitioner is consulted for the first session.

Cranial Osteopathy

William Garner Sutherland who was an American osteopath and a disciple of Andrew Still developed in the 1930s a distinct branch of osteopathy called cranial osteopathy. This discipline uses gentle techniques to manipulate the bones of the skull which are able to move slightly. Inside the skull the brain is surrounded by cerebrospinal fluid (CSF) which flows down the spine covering the spinal cord and the base of the spinal nerves. The brain is held in place by membranes and connective fluid which extends down to the sacrum (part of the pelvis).

Practitioners think the CSF is pumped through the spinal canal by a rhythmic pulsing called the cranial rhythmic impulse. If the bones move normally the rhythm will be normal (6-12 beats per minute), if they are disturbed, for instance when a baby is born the rhythm is interrupted. If there is an irregularity this will be felt by exerting gentle pressure on the skull; the irregularities can be restored by gentle manipulation of the bones.

A cranial osteopath will;
- take a case study like any other osteopath
- ask for details about falls or head injuries
- undertake a full physical assessment.

The treatment is very gentle and relaxing and suitable for babies, children and those adults who do not want a full osteopathy treatment. It is possible that symptoms will worsen over the next couple of days (the 'healing process'); if this happens consult the practitioner. Childhood conditions such as glue ear and breathing problems and in adults; migraine, dizziness, neuralgia, sinus problems, tinnitus and head and neck injuries are some of the ENT conditions which can be helped by this form of osteopathy.

Reflexology

Reflexology has its roots in the ancient Egypt, India and China and in Africa and North America. It was taken up and made real progress in the USA in the 19th century when Dr William Fitzgerald became interested in the European idea of zone therapy where the body is divided into ten vertical zones and by pressing on one part of a zone a positive effect could be felt in another part of the zone. Dr Fitzgerald's ideas were shared with a colleague, Dr Joe Riley and through him to Eunice Ingham, a physiotherapist. Ingham renamed zone therapy as reflexology and she drew the charts showing the feet reflex zones. She also produced the charts of the hands reflex zones as the hands can be used if the feet can not be used for any reason.

Reflexology works on the principle that by pressing a point on the foot (or hand) it will stimulate a positive response in the part of the body/organ/system to which it is thought to correspond. A muscle or organ can have a reflex action when it is activated by energy from a point of stimulus in the body i.e. the foot (or hand).

A reflexologist can ease tension, reduce inflammation and stimulate bodily circulation. These results are achieved by stimulating the nerve endings in the foot and thence stimulating the autonomic nervous system which is connected to all parts of the body. As the body and the foot which reflects it are divided into vertical zones it is thought that a problem in an organ can also affect other structures in the same zone. Cross reflexes mean that if the left leg is hurt the left arm reflex can be treated.

The shape of the feet mirror the shape of the body so it is relatively straightforward for a reflexologist to identify which part of the foot to treat from the symptoms described by the client. For instance if the right eye is sore the correct reflex is under the first and second toes on the right foot.

The reflexologist will use a number of techniques including thumb walking, finger walking, rotating, flexing and relaxation massage strokes.

A reflexologist will;
- take a case study
- ask about work and leisure activities
- enquire about general lifestyle
- explain about the treatment and what effects to expect
- treat both feet (or hands) on a couch or reclining chair with oil, cream or powder having cleansed them first
- deduce past medical events from the reflex reactions
- try to break up crystalline deposits under the skin which feel like grains of sand - these represent energy blockage in the corresponding part of the body
- allow the client to relax at the end of the treatment session
- offer some self help advice to the client to be followed before the next treatment.

There are a number of effects which could be experienced by the client including crying, laughter, depression, elation, headaches and bloating. These show that emotional or physical changes have been instigated by the therapist.

Most ENT conditions can be treated with reflexology. The following reflexes will be concentrated on depending on the condition being treated - the eyes, mouth, nose, sinuses, shoulder, neck, spine, lymph glands, ileo-coecal valve, adrenals, kidney, pineal, pituitary, thymus and spleen reflexes.

Shiatsu and Acupressure

Shiatsu

Shiatsu originated in Japan and is the successor to an older therapy called Anma which primarily used rubbing and pressing techniques. In the 20th century Anma techniques were combined with osteopathic and chiropractic type movements to develop Shiatsu (which is Japanese for 'finger pressure').

Shiatsu practitioners use their elbows, palms, feet and knees as well as fingers to apply pressure on specific tsubo (Japanese for 'little pot') pressure points along the 12 main body meridians. This could be compared to acupuncture without needles and with a shared philosophy, diagnostic techniques and pressure points. Usually the practitioner works through clothing although some parts such as the arms and feet will be exposed briefly. There may also be manipulation of joints and stretching to open up meridians by releasing energy ('ki') blockages and to stimulate the various organs or systems.

The practitioner will use several strands of diagnosis - looking, touching, asking and intuition. A case study will be taken and in most cases the treatment is carried out with the client lying on a large mat so that both the client and practitioner feel 'grounded'.

The treatment works on both a superficial and a deep level and whilst some people feel better after the treatment, others will feel unwell for about 24 hours and this is due to what therapists call a 'healing process' which means that toxins are being released by the body and the ki is being unblocked. The symptoms can include fatigue, bowel changes and headaches - although these changes can be worrying try to remain calm but ring the practitioner after 24/48 hours for reassurance and advice. A 'healing process' can be associated with any therapy and this is something which should be explained to the client prior to the first treatment.

Headaches and migraines, tonsillitis, laryngitis, rhinitis, catarrh (overproduction of mucus in the nose and respiratory tract), colds and ear infections are ENT conditions that can be helped by shiatsu and acupressure.

Acupressure

Acupressure works in similar ways to shiatsu but the big difference is that only finger and thumb pressure on tsubos with additional massage strokes along the meridians are used. Acupressure is usually incorporated into a shiatsu treatment although it is the basis for seated clothed upper body massage which is often called 'On site massage' which is becoming increasingly popular at the workplace and in public places like exhibitions, conferences and shopping malls.

ENT problems which are treated by acupressure have similar results as those which are treated by shiatsu.

CHAPTER 10: SELF HELP AND USEFUL ORGANISATIONS

Introduction

So far in this book we have examined the structure of the different parts of the ear and inner head, how they function, conditions which can affect them and treatments to hopefully improve their situation. In chapter 6 we touched on measures an individual can adopt to prevent problems and in this chapter we are going to further examine ways by which an individual can help him/herself together with the role of useful organisations which can be contacted for assistance.

Self Help

Although most treatments discussed so far have been in the realm of conventional medicine and allied skills there has already been some mention of complementary therapies, notably the ear candling treatment, and self help for both prevention and treatment of conditions. For example whilst divers should think hard before going to depth if suffering from a middle ear infection, no-one should push anything into the outer ear canal in order to remove wax.

Diet and Nutrition

Diet is undoubtedly an important factor in the cause of many problems such as migraines or snoring. Before making any great changes to any diet it is advisable that an individual contact a properly qualified and insured practitioner to avoid any serious consequence which may be brought about. It is advisable to consult a properly qualified and insured practitioner of any therapy.

Helpful Organisations

Often because of the nature of many conditions, especially those affecting hearing, people feel isolated with their problem. There have been a number of associations and charities set up which can offer specific advice for example on helpful devices which are available and support to the affected individual often through the contents of their regular journals or newsletters. These organisations are often run by understanding individuals who may suffer from the condition with which they are concerned. They often act as pressure groups and advisors to politicians and other interested parties The contact details of a number of these organisations are shown later in the book.

Devices which can be used

There are a large number of devices and systems which can be employed to reduce the effects of many of the problems associated with many of the conditions afflicting the 'ear and inner head environments'; possibly the most commonly known are the different types of hearing aid which can be worn. These devices and systems have made life much more tolerable and the process of living less embarrassing for many sufferers of ear, nose and throat (and associated) conditions.

Ear, Nose, Throat and Associated Conditions

We will look at the following conditions and see how the four categories of advice - self help; complementary therapies and other treatments; diet and nutrition; and helpful organisations can assist a sufferer of a condition. In some instances two or more of the categories may overlap.

The conditions are;
- **hearing problems and ear infections**
- **Patulous Eustachian Tube**
- **balance problems**
- **tinnitus**
- **Ménière's Disease**
- **dizziness**
- **vertigo**
- **sinusitis**
- **rhinitis**
- **snoring**
- **Sleep Apnoea**
- **headaches**
- **migraines**
- **motion sickness**
- **neuralgia**
- **Bell's Palsy**
- **colds and flu**
- **Laryngitis**
- **Tonsillitis**
- **Adenoidal conditions.**

Hearing Problems and ear infections

Prevention of hearing loss

It is important to protect the ears and prevent their damage. If hearing loss has occurred the hearing which remains can be enhanced and further deterioration should be prevented for as long as possible. There are aids of all types which can assist a hearing impaired or profoundly deaf person whether mechanical or of a 'doggy' nature as provided by the Hearing Dogs for Deaf People charity.

If earrings or studs are to be fitted to the pinna good quality metal should be used and the hole should be made in sterile conditions - these precautions should prevent infection. If contact sports such as rugby or American football are played or sports undertaken which carry the risk of a fall from height or at speed, for example horse riding, head protection should be worn.

Children should be deterred from putting beads or seeds into the ear canal. If objects including insects have to be removed from the canal this should be done by a medical practitioner. The outer ear canal should not be poked by any implement to clear out the cerumen wax which is a protective mechanism.

Protective ear wax (cerumen) is produced in response to different stimuli and causes. Certain cultures have a history of cleansing the canal by using a natural substance such as warmed olive oil. It is thought that wax and mucous production is stimulated by the ingestion of dairy products and fatty foods; these ingredients in the diet could be reduced although questions such as the need for calcium and prevention of osteoporosis have to be considered.

The World record holder (at 12. 02. 2002) for hair sprouting from his ears was Mr B D Tyagi of Bhopal, India whose hair measured 10 cms. While this is quite an achievement it would mean that it is difficult for water to drain from his ears after they had been washed. It is recommended that ear hair is kept short and tidy so that water and soap/shampoo/shaving foam residue can be easily removed from the ears. After having a grommet or drainage tube implanted in the ear, protective ear plugs should be used.

Many people who work and play in noisy, dirty or dusty environments or who come in contact with dirty water could consider wearing suitable ear protection in the form of ear plugs or ear defenders (muffs). There are a number of different types available for different purposes. A diver should not wear ear plugs if he/she also wears a tight fitting hood. If telephone head sets are worn, for instance by workers in call centres, they should be cleaned regularly especially if they are shared by more than one person.

The other part of the ear which is the location of conductive hearing loss is the middle ear which is affected by damage to the ossicle bones and different infections including glue ear which is especially prevalent in children. A child's Eustachian tube is shorter and straighter than an adult's and it also can be affected by enlarged adenoids. The best way of reducing problems in this area is to strengthen the immune system by following a good diet and adopting a healthy lifestyle. Preferred foods include; organic fresh food, raw or lightly cooked food, whole grain products, vegetables, fruit, fish, poultry, pulses, polyunsaturated fats and vegetable oils, and rice/pasta/potatoes if filling foods are liked. Obviously food intolerances have to be taken into account.

The cochlea in the inner ear and the acoustic nerve leading to the brain are the two areas where sensorineural hearing loss happens. As the endolymphatic fluid in the cochlea has a high sodium content it is a good idea to reduce intake of this mineral, in the form of salt, in the diet. A high level of salt intake is also not good for blood pressure or the kidneys. It is interesting that a complication of strep. tonsillitis can be nephritis which is an inflammation of the kidney(s). In Traditional Chinese Medicine, ear problems are thought to be associated with imbalances in the kidney meridian; in Auriculotherapy the outer ear is thought to resemble either a foetus or a kidney.

'Damage to the delicate hearing 'hair' cells in the cochlea is the most common form of deafness in the UK' (from the Bulletin of the Defeating Deafness hearing research charity, London) and while the hairs cannot be replaced one of the major causes of damage - exposure to loud noise - can be reduced by using ear protection (which can be hidden and unobtrusive); and by not risking damage e.g. by not going to too many loud music concerts or not sitting for too long plane spotting under flight paths at the perimeter of major airports.

Although hearing damage can be instantaneous, most damage tends to result from repeated exposure. Regular breaks should be taken from prolonged loud noise - 10 minutes every hour for example would allow for a cup of tea in a parked car while plane spotting.

Ears should be given time to recover from excessive noise. Exposure to 100 dB for two hours requires at least 16 hours rest to avoid permanent hearing damage. Examples of common noise levels will include;
- nightclubs and pop concerts - 120 dB
- classical concerts - up to 100 dB
- films - peak levels up to 120 dB.

Music fans should try to avoid standing too close to speakers or other noise sources at music concerts or 'raves' and in appropriate venues consider wearing discreet ear plugs. Musicians whether they are playing electric heavy metal music or loud classical symphonies should also take care of their hearing.

Aids to help those with partial or total hearing loss

There are a number of mechanical aids which are available to help people with partial or total hearing loss. As well as mechanical aids which can be worn, other forms of mechanical aid can be used in the home, work of leisure environments.

It is essential for deaf people to take part in ordinary activities - a visit to the doctor, chatting with family or colleagues or a job interview. It is important to be able for them to focus on the content and not the communication.

Deaf people can also be helped by such diverse methods such as lip reading, sign language/ 'signing' and the assistance of intelligent, friendly animals such as the dogs which are provided by the charity 'Hearing Dogs for Deaf People' (Registered Charity No: 293358 (England)).

Definitions of levels of hearing loss

There are different levels of someone's hearing loss and these are;

●   **Mild** - there is difficulty following speech in noisy situations
●   **Moderate** - difficulty following speech but can use an amplified telephone
●   **Severe** - rely on lip reading, even with a hearing aid
●   **Profound** - rely on lip reading and may use sign language or speech-to-text.

Types of hearing aids which are available

There are two main types of hearing enhancement which are available to a deaf person - hearing aids or cochlear implants. As we have already seen the assessment, fitting and rehabilitation of those who are suitable for a cochlea implant is both a complicated and expensive procedure and so is not a self help subject. We will therefore in this chapter just look at the other different types of hearing aid which are available and which should be fitted after appropriate medical testing to ensure that the most suitable is used.

Hearing aids

'In the UK two million people use a hearing aid and a further three million people would benefit from one' ('Spring 2002 Bulletin' Defeating Deafness charity, London). Remember wearing one is not a social stigma or something to be embarrassed about.

A hearing aid amplifies sounds so that the wearer can hear them. Their design has been improved over time and they are now more unobtrusive. They are battery operated and are put in or around the ear.

Hearing aids come in different shapes, sizes and types and some are now disposable; they all work on roughly the same principle. The hearing aid which is fitted depends on the hearing loss and what feels comfortable.

All hearing aids have an integral microphone which picks up sound, this sound is processed electronically either by analogue circuits or digitally to make the sound more audible by means of 'signals'. These signals are then passed to a receiver/earphone in the aid where they are converted back into sounds which can be heard. There is also an ear mould, which goes into the ear, tubing and a battery for power.

A hearing aid will not give perfect hearing but it should make sounds louder, help telephone and other conversations, reduce isolation and help with confidence. For those with tinnitus the distinctive sound will hopefully be diminished by the aid. It is important to persevere with the aid until a person gets used to it.

Process of getting a hearing aid

In the UK hearing aids can be supplied free on the National Health Service (NHS) or bought privately. It is wise to firstly get the ears and hearing checked to see if there is hearing loss and if an aid is appropriate. As any hearing difficulty should be investigated, the family doctor (GP) should be approached. This is essential if the hearing aid is to be supplied by the NHS. The GP will refer a patient to an ENT consultant or audiologist at a local hospital. For people over 60, the referral may be direct to the audiology department.

If the hearing aid is being bought privately, a dispenser (often either in a shop on the high street or in a location advertised in the local newspaper) can be visited. He/she will advise if the GP has to be consulted about the hearing loss.

If the hearing aid is being provided by the NHS a patient's hearing will normally be tested by an audiologist in a hospital who will produce an audiogram based on the results of differing frequencies (pitch) and loudness levels which can be heard by the patient. An ENT consultant will beforehand take a case history, including details of family deafness. Because of the pressure on the NHS it is likely that a waiting time to obtain a hearing aid can be up to 18 months.

If an aid is needed, the audiologist will take an impression of the ear to make the ear mould. If hearing aids are offered for both ears it may be a good idea to take up the offer. It may take a few weeks for the aid to be ready and the audiologist may have to adjust it and offer guidance on its use and care.

If the aid is digital there may be a need to return to have it fine tuned and there should be a follow up appointment to see how things are going. A hearing aid normally lasts about five years and during this time hearing may change (normally deteriorate) and a more powerful one may be needed.

If a hearing aid is being bought privately it should be from a dispenser who is qualified, or in supervised training with, and registered with the Hearing Aid Council. Hearing is tested and there should be a period to try it/them out. It is usually quicker to get an aid privately and some types of aid are only available privately. The cost of the aid can vary from £300 to £3,000 and the purchaser has to pay for new batteries and other items. The aid should be insured against loss, theft or damage.

Because the subject of hearing aids and questions such as which are the most suitable for the individual is complicated it may be advisable for a potential user, or parent of a child, to contact charities such as the RNID or the National Deaf Children's Society who can give advice and issue informative literature. Throughout the country there are local organisations who give talks on hearing concerns, hearing aids, lipreading skills and other related matters. In Shropshire where the author lives, the Effective Hearing Programme is organised by the Sensory Resource Service at the Disability Resource Centre, Shrewsbury.

Types of hearing aid

There are many types of hearing aid - analogue or digital. Digital types are newer and have an integral tiny computer to process sound, they also have inbuilt compression. Although digital hearing aids are easily available privately they are only now becoming more available through the NHS within the UK.

The types of hearing aid available are;

- **Behind the ear (BTE) aids** - the most common type and most people who get one through the NHS get one of these
- **In the ear (ITE) and in the Canal (ITC) aids** - not usually for severe hearing loss or for small ear canals
- **Body-worn aids** - a small box is connected to the earphone and ear mould. Not often used but can be very powerful
- **Bone conduction hearing aids** - for people with conductive hearing loss or who cannot wear a conventional aid
- **CROS/BiCROS aids** for people with no hearing in one ear; **CROS** feeds sound to the good ear, **BiCROS** aids amplify sound from both sides and feeds it to the ear that has some hearing
- **Disposable hearing aids** - suitable for those with only a mild to moderate hearing loss. They normally last (about 6 weeks) as long as the battery; early results have not always proved to be successful
- **Waterproof and water-resistant aids** - have a thin membrane to stop water entering the ear. Waterproof for swimming and water- resistant for other water sports
- **Bone Anchored Hearing Aids** - this type is mainly for people who cannot wear ordinary hearing aids because of discharge and who suffer from unilateral hearing loss. The aid is fitted surgically by screwing it, using a titanium screw, to the skull on the affected side; sound is transmitted via bone to the normal side and the perception is that sound is heard on the affected side! The aid which costs about £2,000 can be taken off when swimming, sleeping, bathing etc.

Use of a hearing aid

As soon as someone gets a hearing aid he/she should practice using it and its controls and also check that the ear mould feels comfortable. There is usually a switch or small press button controls with 'O' (off)/ 'M' (microphone)/ 'T' positions and also a volume control which can be adjusted for different situations and noisy environments. If the aid does not have an 'O' position the battery door will have to be opened slightly to switch it off. When choosing a hearing aid it is advantageous if it has a 'T' (telecoil) position. Remember that a battery has a limited life so at the first sign of it losing power buy a spare.

The importance of the 'T'(telecoil) position on the hearing aid

Use of the 'T' position allows the hearing aid to pick up sound from specially designed external listening equipment (an induction loop) which transfers sound direct to the hearing aid cutting out background noise. If the system has been installed in public places such as theatres or at post office or bank counters there will be a sign to say this has been done. Sometimes the loop system is not switched on, check!! A loop system can be installed in the home to help listen to a television or sound system and several people can use it at the same time as long as they have a hearing aid or loop listener.

The induction loop

An induction loop is a length of wire which is laid around the edge of a room, usually located at floor level. The ends of the wire are connected to a loop amplifier which is attached to the equipment you want to listen to - either directly or using a microphone (usually attached to the front of the TV loudspeaker grille). The amplifier, which has its own controls for volume and tone, receives the sound signal which is converted into magnetic waves by the loop. When the waves reach the hearing aid or loop listener they are converted back to sound which can be heard. A big advantage of using a Portable Loop, Neckloop or Headphone set is that these types of equipment have their own volume controls so that the person with hearing loss can adjust the volume to his/her comfort level, independent of the TV volume - to the relief of anyone else who may have been blasted by an excessive noise level.

Headphone sets have the advantage of being portable and can have a good quality of sound. They are mainly suitable for those people whose hearing loss is not severe; hearing aid users have to temporarily remove them.

Other equipment to help hearing include telephones described as 'hearing aid compatible' with a type of built-in loop in the earpiece of the headset and also sound amplifiers for telephones, television, music and conversations with or without a hearing aid.

A device called a loop listener allows someone without a hearing aid to be able to use the loop. Various types of loop listener are available as a small box with plug-in headphones.

Cleaning the hearing aid

Because part or all of the hearing aid is positioned in the ear canal it is important that it is kept clean to avoid infection and damage. Because of the different available types of aid cleaning methods vary. When a user obtains the aid advice on cleaning should be given verbally and in writing. Some aids have tubing and if this hardens the aid will not work well and if it splits the aid will whistle. This type of aid should come with spare tubing and the user should be shown how to replace it or know where to get the hearing aid retubed e.g. in clinics or by volunteers.

Problems with hearing aids

Size
Many people do not wear a hearing aid because they erroneously think that they are all bulky devices possibly remembering the large 'body worn' devices. Modern aids have been dramatically reduced in size mainly due to digital chip technology, smaller batteries and other spin offs from the mobile phone industry and the recording industry's better understanding of sound reproduction. A new model (The GN ReSoundAir) which is being trialled in the UK and which has already been successful in Denmark, for those with mild to moderate hearing loss, weighs only nine grams is less than an inch long and 0.2 inches wide. Its small transparent tube, which replaces the traditional sound tube and earplug, will not block the ear so while high pitched sounds are amplified other sounds are heard naturally.

Problems with the 'In the Ear' and 'In the Canal' types are that they are so small they can get lost and also because they do not have an ear mould they do not fit as well and this can lead to noises such as whistling or squeaking. They are only suitable for a mild/moderate hearing loss.

Malfunction
It is obviously worrying if a hearing aid does not work correctly, possible causes include;

- **the aid does not work** - check on the volume level, battery condition, if it is mistakenly set on the 'T' position or the tubing on a BTE type of aid is blocked by condensation
- **whistling or squeaking caused by 'feedback'** which occurs when sound amplified by the hearing aid is fed back into it - possible causes include; ear mould is not in place, excess wax (ask doctor to check), volume too high, ear mould needs to be carefully sealed with Vaseline (used sparingly), check condition of BTE components
- **buzzing** - either the hearing aid has been accidentally turned to the 'T' position or it has developed a fault which needs to be repaired.

    The outer ear canal should be kept dry at all times.

Other Mechanical aids to help deaf people

Having looked in depth at hearing aids and cochlea implants which are worn by deaf people and having touched on the 'T' loop system which can be used in conjunction with many types of hearing aid we can now turn our attention to the different types of equipment which can enhance everyday items which hearing people take for granted. This equipment includes special alarm clocks (ringing), door bells (chimes), baby (cry) speakers or smoke alarms (shrieking). Equipment designed for use by deaf people enhances normal sound by utilising flashing lights or vibrating pads.

Alarm clocks and wristwatch alarms

Some alarm clocks have vibrating pads that can go under a pillow; others have flashing lights which can be next to the bed. Wristwatch alarms can be set to vibrate.

Baby monitors

Baby monitors for deaf people use a flashing light and/or vibrating pad to warn you that a baby is crying.

Doorbells and entry systems

If a louder doorbell, chime or intercom is not the answer then there are different systems available using flashing or dimming lights which tell a deaf person that a visitor is at the front door. Radio waves using a receiver and a transmitter can send signals all around the house to work lights in all rooms.

Smoke alarms

Smoke alarms which register the presence of smoke and a rise in temperature normally emit a very loud warning sound. If these are not adequate, alarms can use added vibrations or flashing strobe lights.

Telephones

Firstly, tone callers can be fitted free; also there can be an increase in the volume of the ringer or to a change to its pitch. The phone can be placed on a hard surface as this will make it ring harder. An extension bell(s) or flashing light(s) could be placed in another room(s). A telephone amplifier could help hear what is being said.

Some phones have an induction coupler incorporated in the handset for people who use a hearing aid with a 'T' setting. This should improve sound clarity with reduced background noise. If a hearing aid is being used it is better to use an analogue phone because digital phones can cause interference with hearing aids. Some shops take back equipment in good condition within a stated time with a price refund; in this way it is possible to try out different models and find which one suits best.

Mobile phones

Technological changes are very fast in this part of the communications market and texting has been a great help for deaf people. They have a number of ring tones available and quite a high ringer volume. Many models can be set to vibrate when they ring and mobile phones are useful in emergencies.

A very recent innovation is the mobile phone which incorporates photographs; while it is necessary for both parties to have compatible phones imaging could be beneficial for deaf people. The texting facility on a mobile phone, especially if it has a querty keyboard has been a great communication help for the Deaf and the general population alike.

Mobile phones in the UK are all digital (not analogue) and like telephones, these can cause interference with hearing aids. Again, all models should be tried out before buying. Listening accessories such as plug in ear and neck hooks can enable the phone to be used more effectively.

Textphones (Minicom)

Textphones are suitable for the severely or profoundly Deaf. They have a small display screen and a keyboard so words can be typed and then read in return. Some models have a voice telephone handset and others can be used with a voice telephone. Many people are now using text on their mobile phones instead.

RNID Typetalk and BT TextDirect

These are two systems whereby a voice telephone can communicate with a textphone. The systems are run by the Royal National Institute for Deaf and Hard of Hearing People (RNID) and funded by British Telecom (BT).

Videophones

Videophones allow seeing, and signing to, people who can be a long distance away - possibly several thousand miles. Although picture quality is good it may be necessary to slow down sign language; it is difficult to lipread unless picture quality is satisfactory. There is also the problem of time delay between sound and picture.

Computers and the Internet

All people, including the Deaf and hard of hearing, can now take advantage of the fast communication links offered on the universal internet using PCs (personal computers), lap tops which can be carried around, notebooks and digital organisers. The cost of all these items has dropped dramatically and they can be bought second hand or used in one of the many internet centres on the high street where a computer is hired for perhaps one hour and e-mails can be accessed and sent worldwide. On the world wide web (www) there are a number of chat rooms where 'friendships' can be started; caution should be exercised to ensure confidential information is not divulged to other people. Many companies now have secure shopping carts where goods can be purchased using credit or debit cards and by this means the purchaser does not have to listen to a sales person or hear instructions.

Fax machines

A fax machine can either share an existing land phone line or have its own dedicated line. It can send and receive letters, drawings or any type of written material to any location in the world. For a hard of hearing, person it would probably be better to have a dedicated phone line otherwise a caller will have to phone to tell the receiver that a fax is about to be sent.

Personal listening equipment

There are many types of equipment which can assist hearing conversation in social or work environments. This equipment includes;

- **conversation aids** - these are small and are best for one to one conversations in a quiet place. They have a microphone, an amplifier to boost speech volume and reproductive equipment e.g. stetoclips, earphones, neckloops or headphones. Whilst many work with radio frequencies some are adapted for listening to induction ('T') loop systems. Advanced systems can be used for distance listening at conferences or meetings. This equipment can help hear sound more clearly from the TV, video, radio or any type of sound system.

- **loop or infrared systems** - as we have seen these can be used both at home and in public places such as banks and theatres. A loop system can be set up with a microphone to help hearing aid users hear conversations in noisy places. An alternative infrared system needs a transmitter and an infrared receiver and no cables get in the way. There is a range of 12 m but visual contact has to be maintained with the transmitter. Strong sunlight can interfere with infrared systems so they should be kept away from direct sunlight.

Subtitles on television and at the cinema

Many television programmes have subtitles to assist the Deaf and hard of hearing; in the UK subtitles are on teletext page 888. Programmes written specially for Deaf and hard of hearing people are 'Deafview' on Channel 4, teletext page 467 and 'Read Hear' on BBC 2 on teletext page 640.

Some pre-recorded DVDs and videotapes also have subtitles. Foreign films often have sub titles instead of being dubbed into the mother tongue language.

An aerial booster may be needed to ensure that the teletext subtitles are clear.

Equipment in cars for drivers and passengers

There is a wide range of equipment which is designed to help Deaf and hard of hearing drivers and passengers to enjoy a journey more, including;
- loop systems for listening to conversations and the radio/CD/cassette
- car radios that display information in a text form e.g. traffic jams
- visual car alarms
- satellite navigational road maps
- products to help park the car
- equipment to tell you to turn off indicators if they have been left on.

Communication services which are available

Having looked at many of the mechanical aids which are available to help Deaf, deafened and hard of hearing people ('deaf' people) we can now examine some of the services which are available in the UK to help people communicate. The RNID in London has an excellent information line which can advise people about what is available and other aspects such as costs and servicing.

Lip reading and sign language

Before looking at external services which are available it should be said that many 'deaf' people use lip reading to understand hearing people better and communicate together through a system of sign language.

Lip reading

If lip reading is being used, the hearing person who is speaking should try to make things easier for the listener by;
- facing directly towards the listener
- speaking slowly and clearly
- using words comprehensible to the listener.

British Sign Language (BSL) is the preferred language of approximately 70,000 'Deaf' people for whom English is a secondary language; over 100,000 hearing people can also use it. BSL is a visual/spatial language which has its own grammatical rules using hand shapes, hand movements and facial expressions. BSL can be learnt at many local Adult Education Centres, whose contact details are to be found in local telephone directories or libraries. Alternatively, a SAE could be sent to the Council for the Advancement of Communication with Deaf People (CACDP) which is the national board for BSL examinations.

Available communication services for Deaf people

Using outside interpreters/support workers costs money but for the Deaf or Deafblind costs should be covered by the government and its agencies. Owing to demand, bookings for interpreters should be made as soon as possible and if a lengthy assignment is planned two experts should be engaged. The interpreters are bound by a code of ethics that includes impartiality and confidentiality.

Interpreters/support workers engaged will be in the following specialisms;
- BSL/English interpreters (including video interpreting)
- Communication support workers
- Deafblind interpreters and communicator guides
- Electronic notetakers
- Speech-to-text reporters
- Lipspeakers
- Notetakers.

BSL/English interpreters

These interpreters are used by Deaf people whose preferred language is BSL when they are communicating in writing or speaking with a hearing person. The interpreter should have completed approved training and be registered with a professional body such as CACDP or ASLI. The interpreter will need a break about every 30 minutes and is usually booked for at least two hours and specific costs and other information, will be confirmed when the booking is made. There are about 800 fully qualified interpreters throughout the country and coverage varies greatly. A problem for many people wanting to progress through the stages of training to become a BSL interpreter is not only the availability and fees for courses but often travelling and accommodation costs have to be funded in a large part by the individual.

Video interpreting
Several organisations, including the RNID, offer a video interpreting scheme. This has advantages if the meeting is short or there are difficulties in booking an interpreter at short notice. A videophone and ISDN2 line are prerequisites to booking a video interpreter.

Communication support workers
These workers support Deaf people, usually in an educational setting and are the link between the client student and the tutor and other students. Their skill levels vary and they may use BSL or SSE (Sign Supported English).

Deafblind interpreters and communicator guides
Deafblind interpreters and communicator guides liaise between deafblind people and hearing or sighted people. They use a variety of aids including BSL, hands-on-signing, the Block Alphabet, the Deafblind Manual Alphabet or speech-to-Braille.

The interpreters work in more formal settings such as training courses while the communicator guides work more informally e.g. they can help write a letter or go out shopping with a client.

Electronic notetakers
Electronic notetakers/operators work with Deaf people who are able to read English as all notes are typed in English; they can also assist hearing people who want to communicate with Deaf people.

The notetakers/operators type a summary of what is being said on a computer and this information is then projected on to a screen. The words are less than with speech-to-text but it is less accurate.an ordinary computer with software is needed but a more sophisticated system is possible using special software such as RNID SpeedText which uses two laptops linked to their own screen. Replies can be typed which can be read to hearing people.

Palentype and Speech - to - Text reporters

While Speech - to- text reporting is suitable for Deaf people who are comfortable reading English at high speed with a conventional querty keyboard being used a Palentype reporter uses a special keyboard. Every word is typed that is spoken by a speaker; these spoken words are then projected on to a large screen or several small screens. Speech - to - text is not as complete as Palentype as it focuses more on core learning.

Lipspeakers
Lipspeakers work with deaf people who prefer to communicate through lipreading and speech. Hearing people can also use lipspeakers to help them communicate with deaf people as lipspeakers can repeat what lipreaders have said.

Lipspeakers repeat what is said, without using their voice so that they can be lipread easily. They can also use natural gestures and facial expression and fingerspelling if requested to do so. Level three lipspeakers shorten speech that is too fast to lipread without losing its meaning.

Notetakers

A notetaker works with Deaf people who are comfortable reading English. They work at meetings, courses or at other events. The notetakers write notes in a way which is suitable for the Deaf reader.

Often a notetaker is used in conjunction with another professional such as an interpreter or lipspeaker because it may be difficult to take notes while watching a lipspeaker or sign language interpreter. Notetakers may specialise in a particular subject so that he/she is familiar with certain topics.

The Hearing Dogs for Deaf People Charity

This registered charity (No: 293358 (England)) whose modern headquarters are at Princes Risborough, Buckinghamshire has a simple and inspiring mission statement: 'To offer greater independence, confidence and security to deaf people by providing dogs trained to alert them to chosen everyday sounds'.

The scheme, which started in 1982, to train selected dogs to respond to everyday sounds like telephones and doorbells and danger signals such as smoke alarms both helps their deaf human owners to stay independent and also boost confidence by keeping them safe. As dogs, they provide warmth and companionship and also help break down barriers and isolation that many Deaf people, especially, experience.

The scheme was based on similar programmes which were up and running in different parts of the United States. It received support from different quarters including the RNID, a national newspaper, a pet food manufacturer, the British Veterinary Association, Pro-Dogs animal charity, an American insurance company and a large construction company.

In South Africa, there is a similar scheme for training dogs that will help Deaf and hard of hearing people. It is organised by SAGA (the South Africa Guide Dogs Association).

Selection of recipients

The charity has a number of criteria for selecting people for a hearing dog;
● they have a severe, profound or total hearing loss
● they can show a real need for the help of a hearing dog i.e. they live alone, spend a lot of time alone or with another deaf or disabled person(s)
● they are physically and financially able to care for a dog and also like them
● they must be 18 years of age or over.

Having received an application form and recent audiological assessment, a representative of the Charity carries out an interview at the applicant's home before a final decision is made.

183

Selection of dogs

Most selected dogs come from rescue centres or similar backgrounds and vary from scruffy mongrels to pedigrees. They range in size from small to medium and aged from six weeks to three years. The dog must be friendly and outgoing, good tempered, intelligent and inquisitive.

Training and placing a selected dog

The steps for training a selected dog are;

1.   spending a few months in the home of a socialiser, who is a volunteer member of the public who provides temporary care and basic training to the Charity's new recruits. They also introduce the dog to a wide variety of environments and people of all ages. Constant assessments are made during socialisation

2.   dogs are then brought into the Charity's kennels and more assessments are made with a particular recipient in mind. There is a veterinary examination and castration/spaying of unneutered dogs. A photograph is sent to the recipient who meets the dog and its trainer

3.   the advanced soundwork stages of training takes 16 weeks in the purpose built training centres, which are units built as houses resembling a future home for a dog. The dog is taught the sounds it will alert his future Deaf owner to; household sounds such as the telephone, doorbell and alarm clock and danger signals like the smoke alarm. The dog will alert to household sounds by finding and touching the trainer with a paw and then lead him/her to the source of the sound. For danger signals, the dog will alert in the same way, but instead of leading to the sound source, he will lie down in a special way to indicate danger. The dog is also taught basic obedience exercises - 'come', 'sit', 'down', 'stay' and also to walk calmly by the left side of the trainer. Spoken commands are reinforced with hand signals, as some recipients may not have clear speech. The socialisation training is also continued by the trainer who takes the dog out for walks to become familiar with traffic and other environmental noises

4.   at the end of the dog's four month course the recipient comes to one of the training centres for five days where he/she works daily with the new dog and trainer where alert responses to sounds are transferred from the trainer to the recipient. Advice about feeding and other aspects of general care are given and visits are made to public places. The recipient and dog then return home at the end of the week, and the dog will wear a Hearing Dogs' burgundy 'In Training' working jacket

5.   starting on the Tuesday of the following week one of the Charity's placement officers will make daily visits for three days to help, give encouragement, build confidence and practise sound responses and obedience with recipient and dog. The dog is registered with a reputable veterinary practice

6.   after the first week, daily reports are sent to the Centre by the recipient to maintain contact. Three to four weeks later the placement officer will visit for a further two days. For a further two months contact is maintained by telephone or letter from the trainer or placement officer to make sure that the dog and recipient are suited, happy and working well together

7.   a final assessment is made after the recipient has had the dog for three months. A successful recipient will receive an identification certificate for the newly qualified hearing dog, a new burgundy qualified Hearing Dogs' jacket, collar and Hearing Dogs' for Deaf People lead slip cover. The identification allows them to take their dog into shops, to travel on public transport and receive a variety of concessions currently available to assistance dogs (similar to those who help blind people)

8.   there is a support service for all owners of a hearing dog and they will be visited at least once a year to ensure standards are maintained and that dog and owner continue to work well together.

As at February 2004 the Charity has placed over 1,000 hearing dogs with deaf people in the UK. The aim is to place approximately 130 dogs each year; there is a waiting time of approximately one year. If an owner dies the Charity will find a home for the dog to continue its job. The Charity will re-home dogs which do not make the grade as a Hearing dog. A milestone in the Charity's progress was reached in November 2003 when Labrador cross Roddy became the first ever fully qualified hearing and guide dog. Roddy, and his owner were trained by the Charity in conjunction with Guide Dogs for the Blind charity. His success signals a brighter future for more deaf-blind people.

Ear infections

While infections can affect any part of the ear, it is the outer and middle ear infections which can be influenced by an individual.

The outer ear

The outer ear canal can be damaged by scratching it with implements such as cotton buds and this is an entry point for infection to develop so nothing 'smaller than an elbow' should be poked in the ear.

Water should be prevented from entering the canal by wearing bathing or shower hats or ear plugs. Regular swimmers should dry their ears with a hairdryer. Bacterial growth can be prevented by putting into the ear either a few drops of equal parts alcohol and white wine vinegar or freshly squeezed lemon juice.

If the ear is prone to produce a lot of wax then the intake of dairy products could be reduced for a period to see if this helps. If production of excess wax is experienced by someone who consumes a lot of yeast- based food and drink such as bread products and beer intake of these items can be reduced for a time to see if the situation improves.

There are many types of ceruminolytic ear drops which are available to help with the problem of excessive ear wax. Most proprietary brands and substances like olive oil are best for softening hardened wax; prepared sodium bicarbonate ear drops have been shown to be best for breaking up the wax. All types of drops should be used with caution and their use should be stopped if any adverse reaction sets in.

Traditional remedies for home made drops include;

● adding olive oil to a mashed clove of garlic which is heated, cooled and strained and then put on cotton wool and placed in the ear canal for a couple of days
● hold half an onion over the ear entrance for thirty minutes
● if there is no discharge or perforated ear drum, squeeze a couple of drops of lemon juice into the ear canal.

A warm hot water bottle or wheat bag can be held against the ear and mastoid process to try to bring relief from an earache.

The middle ear

In the middle ear most infections, especially in children, are due to the malfunction of the Eustachian tube and bacteria which are introduced via the upper respiratory tract. It is important to try to reduce colds and flu by either reducing exposure to other people who may have one and to follow a hygienic regime of washing hands and eating utensils.

The avoidance of drafts and damp places and the consumption of large quantities of vitamin C have not been proved to reduce the incidence of colds and flu. There are a number of over- the- counter preparations available at the chemist or pharmacy for the relief of the symptoms of a cold. The main ingredient is usually a mild analgesic/painkiller such as paracetemol or aspirin which relieves aches and pains. If they include antihistamine or decongestant drugs these should help reduce nasal congestion, Caffeine will act as a stimulant.

Useful information about glue ear can be given by organisations like the RNID, National Deaf Children's Society, Tinnitus Association and many relevant sites on the www. The www is a mine of information about many other ENT conditions and organisations which can be contacted about the various conditions.

Patulous Eustachian Tube

This is a condition where the Eustachian tube remains in the open position instead of being closed. The condition can be treated surgically, but sufferers may be advised to;

● alter medication - oral contraceptives or diuretics
● reduce the intake of caffeine laden drinks including tea, coffee and cola
● increase potassium intake in diet e.g. fruit and vegetables
● reduce fatigue and stress/anxiety levels
● check on an exercise regime
● check on TMJ function
● monitor weight loss
● lie down or place head between knees.

Balance Problems

Balance problems can be divided into uncomfortable dizziness and the more serious condition of vertigo (spinning sensation). Both types of condition have many different causes. A sufferer of either condition could;
- reduce tiredness
- reduce stress
- ensure that any of the causes of anaemia are treated
- reduce hypoglycaemia (low blood sugar level) - this is especially relevant to diabetics
- reduce eye strain and regularly have eyes checked
- if diving, ensure that ascent from depth is carried out correctly
- practice balancing exercises, such as standing on one leg or on a mini trampoline/wobble board. These exercises are best done in a programme (preferably under supervision) devised by a Chartered Physiotherapist or other qualified therapist/trainer.

Tinnitus

Tinnitus is a most insidious condition brought about by damage to either the cochlea part of the inner ear; the auditory nerve or the sound receptor and processing parts of the brain. In chapter 6 we looked at preventative measures - reducing exposure to loud noise at work and during leisure activities, reducing stress, minimal use of aspirin and reducing intake of 'trigger' foods such as chocolate and coffee etc.

Tinnitus often accompanies **sudden sensorineural hearing loss (SSNHL)** when a sufferer goes to bed with normal hearing and wakes up partially or completely deaf in one ear. 95% of new cases of SSNHL have no apparent cause (the remainder being caused by trauma, viruses and measles/German measles). This is a distressing condition with sufferers often unable to go back to work. While most cases recover spontaneously it is vital for all patients to see a specialist urgently to investigate those cases which are treatable and to get support for coping with deafness.

Reduction of tinnitus

There are a number of steps which can be taken to reduce reaction to tinnitus so that it becomes less of a problem. This natural process is known as 'habituation' and habituation therapy (sometimes called Tinnitus Retraining Therapy or TRT) tries to speed up this process. Tools in this therapy include;
- sound therapy - silence is filled by pleasant sound including CDs to make tinnitus sounds less noticeable
- sound generators/tinnitus maskers - can be worn in or behind the ear, resembles or can be combined with a hearing aid and makes a gentle shushing noise. This diverts attention away from the tinnitus
- use of hearing aids - may reduce tinnitus and strain of listening
- use of pillow noise maskers and bedside noise generators
- counselling - helps the sufferer to understand and manage tinnitus
- relaxation and treatment for stress or depression
- medication to help sleeping problems, anxiety, depression or ear infection.

Information and advice

Information and advice about tinnitus, TRT or any other methods of treating it can be obtained from UK charities such as the British Tinnitus Association (BTA) or the Royal National Institute for Deaf and Hard of Hearing People (RNID). These charities offer excellent advice over the telephone and also issue clearly understood literature. They are stockists of relevant merchandise and also encourage local self help groups where members can discuss their condition but also enjoy social activities together. Their details, together with those of other useful organisations are given later in the book.

Importance of sleeping

It is important to use the bed for sleeping (and lovemaking) as watching the television, eating or using a laptop computer will lead the brain to think of these mental activities. Regular sleep patterns are important and if you want to read, go into another room. Waking and getting up should be consistent - do not lie in.

Osteopathic treatments

A cranial osteopath or cranial therapist will check for misalignments of the head and neck which can prevent the lymph glands draining correctly. The osteopath always believes that 'structure governs function'.

Diet
On a dietary note it may be beneficial to try the following;

- reduce mucus forming foods such as full fat milk, cheese and chocolate
- reduce red meat, pies and sausages
- reduce refined foods such as shop- made cakes and pastries which are high in saturated fats and sugar
- increase consumption of fresh vegetables, brown rice and pasta, wholemeal bread, fish and good quality garlic.

Supplements

Two supplements which are applicable are zinc and Ginkgo Biloba. If the sufferer is elderly the herb Ginkgo Biloba should improve the circulation in the ears. As Ginkgo Biloba has blood-thinning properties, great care should be exercised if other blood-thinning/anticoagulant agents such as aspirin or Warfarin are being taken. It may also not be advisable for women who are pregnant or breast feeding.

Massage to the upper neck may be beneficial.

Ménière's Disease

This is a condition which affects people with different individual, or a combination of, symptoms. These include - unilateral or bilateral deafness, tinnitus, 'fullness in the ear', earache, sickness, 'Mal de debarquement' syndrome, vertigo spinning, 'drop' and 'fall' attacks and migraine or headaches which can vary in severity.

Self-help

We have already seen the importance of reducing sodium, salt and caffeine in helping to control the effects of Ménière's Disease; there are a number of other steps a sufferer can take to try to improve his/her condition to augment medical treatment including;

- join a specific organisation, such as the Ménière's Society, UK which can offer assistance in many ways
- plan the day and get up and move about slowly
- listen to relaxing or meditation music
- remove all loose rugs, do not polish floors highly
- go for a daily walk (possibly with the dog), use a walking stick or supermarket trolley for support
- protect the ears in windy conditions and ensure that heavy earrings do not cause discomfort which may lead to vertigo, nausea and headaches
- have eyesight checked regularly and wear the correct glasses and contact lenses
- avoid flickering lights when driving or in the workplace/home and at leisure. Take dark glasses in case there are strobe lights
- watch television or computer screens in a well lit environment (a computer should have a 'refresh rate' over 75 Hz)
- write and complain to television companies and regulators about unnecessary intrusive background noise and music
- avoid having moving objects in the peripheral vision - movements out of the corner of the eye
- limit the length of time looking through binoculars, telescopes or magnifying glasses
- wear flat shoes, cool clothing and have extra items available which will reduce stress e.g. gloves and hats if the weather becomes cold
- carry plastic bags in case of a sudden bout of sickness
- use a rubber anti-slip mat in the bath or shower and have safety rails to hold throughout the house if balance is poor
- try therapies such as osteopathy, acupuncture, reflexology, ear candling, homeopathy, herbalism, Bowen Technique or Qi Gong
- try reducing intake of dairy products (milk, butter, cheese, cream, yogurt) and substitute with soya, goat or sheep products
- ensure that you do not become dehydrated - drink 2/2.5 litres of water daily
- reduce excessive intake of tea or coffee as these have a diuretic effect
- try taking Ginkgo Biloba, but be careful if drug-thinning drugs such as aspirin are being taken
- peanuts which are rich in nicotinic acid (one of the B vitamins) can be eaten to act as a vasodilator - bear in mind the possibility of a nut intolerance
- swallowing, and chewing sugar free gum, may help symptoms especially 'full ness' of the ear, hearing, tinnitus and vertigo. Chewing should not be done during a major vertigo attack as the situation could be made worse by the induced movement of fluid in the inner ear
- wear a digital or analogue hearing aid if it helps
- install a buzzer in place of a chiming doorbell

- it is important to carry a card stating why a 'drop attack' has occurred (the question of drunkenness can be ruled out) and that the wearer is a Ménière's Disease sufferer
- ensure you have a supply of medication ready - do not run out!
- try taking a quarter of a teaspoon of glace ginger daily to reduce nausea or vomiting - this remedy can be tried to combat any form of travel sickness. If this or any other supplement gives adverse health results stop taking immediately; if in doubt consult a medical practitioner before starting to take it
- wear travel bands, over the acupressure point for nausea and sickness, on the inside of the wrists, to combat travel sickness
- when flying, wear inexpensive silicone 'Ear Planes' to reduce the discomfort of air pressure changes also request salt free meals before flying
- if suffering from noise sensitivity (noise recruitment) try wearing EAR soft earplugs which can be bought in bulk from motorcycle accessory stockists
- when travelling on a boat or ferry improve dizziness by either fixing the eyes on a stationary object such as the horizon or stay close to its centre of gravity such as mid-deck or in the middle of the boat. A vestibular sedative such as Stugeron or travel sickness pills might also help
- try taking Glucosamine Sulphate (which is usually used for joint problems) to combat dizzy spells; a 2 - 3 month period is required to assess improvements
- breathe in ice cold air through the nose while keeping the mouth shut may reduce spinning and nausea
- consider the travel insurance considerations of having Ménière's Disease and if you experience problems contact the Ménière's Society, UK for advice
- if a grommet has been fitted and the feelings of 'fullness' in the ear increases get a GP to check that it has not become blocked.

Help in the workplace

Employers in the UK can receive financial assistance towards the extra costs of employing someone with a disability through the Access to Work programme run by the Employment Service. There is also a duty under the UK Disability Discrimination Act 1995 not to discriminate against disabled people in employment and for employers to make 'reasonable adjustments' for a disabled person or employee if they are at a substantial disadvantage in relation to a non-disabled person. There is a helpful reference web site: http:// www.employers-forum.co.uk/index.htm.

Employers could consider improving the function of people with Ménière's (or with hearing difficulties) with probable productivity benefits by implementing the following;

- work in non - open plan offices or working spaces so sound does not reverberate
- lighting should be good and people should communicate clearly within 4-6 feet to help lip reading
- amplified telephones should help staff with hearing loss
- computers and televisions should have minimum flickering
- all workstations should be ergonomically planned to reduce stress
- ensure that fire alarm systems and test day procedures are known to staff. Visual indicators could be fitted to augment noise alarms
- there should be access to lifts to reduce walking up and down stairs which may trigger dizzy spells
- water dispensers will help reduce thirst and help staff on medication
- employ outside therapists to offer seated massage, reflexology and other forms of treatment and stress management and counselling.

Dizziness

In chapter 5 we looked at the many causes of dizziness. Some of these can be ameliorated with self help measures including;

- reduce tiredness and stress
- anaemia may be helped by eating an iron rich diet (fruit, wholemeal bread, beans, lean meat and green vegetables) or by taking folic acid tablets. Anaemia has many forms and self help measures should follow advice by a medical practitioner
- the risks of hypoglycaemia can be reduced by not missing meals, failure to eat enough carbohydrates or by taking too much exercise. An insulin-dependent diabetic should always carry sugar in the form of sugar lumps or glucose tablets
- eye strain can be reduced by having eyesight checked regularly, wearing correct glasses and contact lenses and working and playing in a 'sight friendly environment'
- wear a telephone headset if using a telephone and computer simultaneously
- reduce the risk of heart attacks and other vascular problems by maintaining a healthy lifestyle - good diet, some exercise, no smoking, moderate (or no) alcohol
- try treatments such as hypnotherapy (anxiety or panic attacks), massage (neck or shoulders), Alexander technique (bad posture), osteopathy or chiropractic (old injury or arthritis).

Vertigo

As vertigo is a symptom of serious conditions such as brain tumours, Ménière's Disease, Multiple Sclerosis and Meningitis self help measures are limited. Sufferers of Ménière's Disease could refer to the section in this chapter dealing with this condition.

Self help can be useful for migraine sufferers and also for those people whose vertigo is triggered by migraine attacks or alternobaric (flying or diving) causes. Migraine will be covered separately later in this chapter.

As vertigo can be triggered by aircraft diving manouevres at altitude too quickly it would be sensible for those travelling in private aircraft not to carry these out deliberately. Commercial airliners normally have smooth phases to their journey and sudden changes in height are usually brought about by adverse weather conditions.

Sub aqua divers can experience vertigo by rising too quickly from depth and care should be taken especially as the 'bends' and damage to the ears can come from incorrect technique.

Vertigo can also be triggered by train and road vehicle passengers staring at objects which pass at speed outside the window. Not staring should reduce the incidence of the condition.

Sinusitis

There are a number of self-help measures which can be taken to prevent and treat sinusitis. The symptoms of sinusitis can be confused with those of rhinitis or other conditions such as cluster headaches and it is important for a medical practitioner to be consulted before embarking on a self- help programme so avoiding making matters worse.

Prevention can be helped by;

● not jumping, diving or swimming in polluted water -this will prevent the water being forced into the sinus cavities (remember there are other risks from polluted water such as Weil's disease)
● regular dental treatment should keep teeth and gums healthy and stop infection spreading to the sinuses up from the mouth
● reduce dairy produce intake to reduce stimulation of mucus production.

Treatment can be;

● the use of non - prescription nasal decongestant drops or sprays available from a pharmacy or chemist
● steam inhalations with the possible addition of eucalyptus or Olbas oils
● the use of a nasal douche containing a saline solution - this is a traditional therapy
● take a warm shower twice a day and expel any excessive mucous through the nose.

Rhinitis

There are different causes of rhinitis and depending on the type the following self help steps can be taken;

- exposure to plants, grasses and trees whose pollen causes an allergic reaction can be reduced by either moving away from their location or by removing them from your garden. It is important to identify the culprit(s) before digging up a prize rose or other specimen plant!
- home and working environments should be cleaned thoroughly to remove, as much as possible, any allergens such as dust, house mites, fur or feathers. There are special vacuum cleaners designed for this task
- fit anti-allergen covers to bed mattresses and pillows
- do not have pets if their fur or feathers cause a reaction
- try taking a puffer called 'Nasaleze' which is non-drowsy and is filled with plant cellulose powder
- eat locally produced honey (possibly in capsule form) daily - this is a homeopathic remedy to build up resistance to allergens
- take a homeopathic remedy like Country Life's 'Aller-Max' which includes stinging nettles which counters histamine, vitamin C and quercetin
- take a daily dose of the herb Butterbur
- drink mixed cod liver oil with fruit juice - this is a natural anti-inflammatory which protects the membranes in the eyes, nose and throat
- drink a daily ginger tonic drink (ginger/water/honey) every morning on an empty stomach - mucus production will be decreased and excess mucus liquefied
- eliminate dairy products for three months and use a substitute soya or rice milk
- eliminate any foods which may cause a reaction
- stop smoking and stay out of polluted atmospheres
- try a course of acupuncture or other complimentary therapy before the season starts
- if oral contraceptives or drugs cause a problem consider alternatives.

Snoring

There are a number of causes of snoring and self-help measures include;

- if the snorer is overweight (UK collar size 16 or greater), a weight loss programme and a sensible exercise programme should be followed
- if alcohol is consumed or sleeping pills are taken these should be reduced where possible
- if the snorer is a smoker this habit should be stopped; if cessation is not possible the last cigarette/cigar/pipe should be four hours before going to bed - this recommendation is true for the last alcoholic drink before going to bed
- avoid rich foods e.g. cake or chocolate before bedtime
- try not sleeping on the back as this will reduce the risk of squashing the airway; sew a rubber ball onto the back of a pyjama jacket to make it uncomfortable to lie on the back

- elevate the head by placing extra pillows below the head
- have a steam inhalation before going to bed to reduce nasal congestion
- reduce exposure to allergens such as dust or pet hair as these can cause nasal congestion
- try a homeopathic nasal spray
- take 'Never snore' an all-natural supplement which is GM free suitable for vegans and vegetarians and aims to open the airways and help airflow
- use a mouth spray such as 'Silence' which helps sooth snoring
- wear nasal strips or one of the many mechanical devices that are available to help snorers with different physical characteristics (e.g. mouth open, collapsing nostrils, obstructing tongue)
- join an organisation such as the British Snoring and Sleep Apnoea Society for useful advice and information.

Sleep Apnoea

Although snoring is irritating to all those around who are affected by the noise, sleep apnoea which has several causes is a more serious condition in that the lungs do not receive oxygen and breathing stops for ten seconds or longer at a time. Self help measures include;

- all those actions which relate to snoring as shown previously, especially stop drinking alcohol as it can induce obstructive sleep apnoea in individuals who might otherwise just be snorers.

Headaches

We saw in chapter 8 that there are a number of causes of headaches and while prevention is better than cure the following self help measures can be considered;
- keep a diary of everything that is eaten and drank and of female periods to see if there is a pattern of attacks
- reduce alcoholic drinking to reduce the effect of a 'hangover' - certainly do not mix grape and grain!
- eat regular meals - always breakfast, and then well balanced, little or often
- take breaks, if possible, during long journeys
- improve poor posture to reduce stress on a tight neck or shoulders
- become more relaxed -reduce stress and excitement
- press a thumb against the roof of the mouth for four to five minutes and move the thumb to all the areas - these are good acupressure points
- press the Large Intestine 4 acupressure point on the back of the hand
- have an adequate amount of sleep - not too little, not too much
- have an adequate amount of sex - not too little, not too much!
- reduce intake of 'trigger' foods such as cheese, chocolate, red wine and very cold foods e.g. ice cream or those with stimulating preservatives or additives such as monosodium glutamate or nitrates/nitrites. Cheese which is low in tyramine such as cottage cheese or Feta is better than those which are high in tyramine such as Cheddar and Parmesan

- eat a few strawberries as they contain organic salicylates which mimic the action of aspirin
- use (preferably extra virgin) olive oil regularly because it contains a compound (olecanthal) that mimics the pain relieving action of ibuprofen
- reduce intake of monosodium glutamate (E621) which is found in Chinese dishes and many other foods including some nibbles, pies, tinned and dried soups, beefburgers, sausages and dips
- mix a teaspoon of honey with half a teaspoon of garlic juice
- take feverfew (Tanacetum parthenium) - fresh, dried or in tablet form
- if the headache is caused by sinusitis slowly sniff some horseradish juice
- rub the forehead and temples with wide pieces of lemon rind
- have eyes tested regularly and wear correct glasses and contact lenses
- ensure there is adequate lighting at work and during leisure
- do not be exposed to excessive or prolonged noise levels
- have regular dental checks to reduce toothache
- try to avoid sinusitis and earaches
- try to avoid the risk of head injury or concussion by wearing correct head protection
- reduce, or preferably give up, smoking as this may lead to cluster headaches
- try to reduce the risk of high blood pressure - reduce salt, red meat, certain fats, smoking, alcohol and take regular exercise and follow a good diet including drinking plenty of water (to reduce the risk of dehydration)
- try applying 'Migraine Ice' drug free cooling therapy patches, which are available from pharmacies, to the forehead, neck or temples where the pain is worse
- take analgesics but do not become dependent on them and check that they will not affect other medication being taken.

Migraines

- The self help methods listed for headaches could also be considered by migraine sufferers.

- The wearing of a correct oral device by someone suffering from TMJ/jaw joint dysfunction might also be a help. This condition can be characterised by a clicking or sticking jaw, difficulty in swallowing or grinding of teeth.

- Research carried out by M. Grossman and H.Schmidrams at the University of Munich indicated that intake of 50mg of the herb Butterbur Petasin extract twice daily for three months markedly reduced the incidence of attacks and there were fewer side effects like nausea and sensitivity to noise. Other research in a clinical trial in Germany and the USA into the use of this herb is also encouraging.

- Have the heart checked for a common harmless anomaly called a Patent Foramen Ovale (PFO) which may be linked to migraine

- A sufferer can get useful information and advice from either the Migraine Action Association or The Migraine Trust.

Motion Sickness

In chapter 8 we looked at the causes of motion/travel sickness and how it can be prevented; it may be useful to reiterate some of the self help measure which can ameliorate this unpleasant condition;

- carry out tasks or entertainment which minimise eye and head movement
- have good environmental conditions - heating, lighting and ventilation
- passengers should be located in a position of least vehicle oscillation such as in the middle of a coach or ferry
- use a headrest and lie down on a bed/bunk (if possible)
- do not follow movement of vehicles or stare at objects passing by outside a window
- look at a point on the horizon if this helps
- do not read if this triggers the condition
- light consumption of food and drink prior to the journey - minimal amount during the journey and try not to travel on a full stomach
- have a sick bag ready but then forget about the possibility of sickness during the journey
- try an alternative homeopathic remedy such as root ginger, Rhus Tox or Tabacum under the direction of a qualified homeopath
- wear a strap on the Nei-Kuan acupressure point just above the wrist
- take anti- travel sickness pills before the journey or wear patches on the skin. Some drugs cause drowsiness and increase the effects of alcohol
- do not take the journey if it is not necessary.

Neuralgia

There are only a few self help measures which can be taken against this condition, these include;

- trying to minimise the risk of facial injury at work and leisure
- protecting the face from wind and cold
- trying to minimise the risk of sinusitis and dental problems
- using hot and cold compresses on an affected area
- considering complementary therapies such as acupuncture, biofeedback and ear candling

Bell's palsy

As well as using the self help methods for neuralgia a sufferer of Bell's palsy could consider the following;

- massage the face gently with a moisturiser
- use a muscle stimulator
- exercise the facial muscles in front of a mirror
- using a finger regularly close the eyelid to moisten the eye
- apply gentle heat e.g. use a wheat bag
- reduce noise on the affected side
- tape the eye closed for sleeping
- wear glasses or a patch to protect the eye from dust
- apply suitable eye drops (artificial tears) to keep the eyeball moist - consult a pharmacist before doing this
- join the Bell's Palsy Association for information and advice.

Colds and flu

People who are in high risk groups should consider having an annual influenza vaccination as this can significantly reduce the risk of hospitalisation or death. Prescription antibiotics do not kill flu or cold viruses and should only be used for rare bacterial complications such as sinusitis or ear infections.

It is better to take preventative measures such as;
● avoiding people who have a cold or flu
● diligent hand washing
● not touching the eyes or nose
● sneezing or coughing into a facial tissue which is immediately disposed of hygienically
● bed rest (to help you and others)
● plenty of fluids
● gargling with warm water
● petroleum jelly for a raw nose
● aspirin (not for children under 16) or paracetemol for headaches or fever
● non-prescription cold remedies including decongestants or cough suppressants may relieve some cold symptoms but can have side effects such as drowsiness, insomnia or upset stomach and should be used with care
● non-prescription antihistamines can help runny nose or watery eyes.

The jury is still out on the effects of taking vitamin C or having steam inhalations; although the steam may temporarily relieve cold congestion symptoms. Too much vitamin C taken over a long period in high doses can be harmful e.g. it may cause severe diarrhoea which is particularly dangerous for the elderly and children.

Laryngitis

Self help measures can include;
● reduce or cease using the voice especially cheering or chanting
● reduce violent coughing by using non-prescription remedies
● stay away from tobacco smoke or other noxious fumes
● reduce alcohol intake
● check that breathing safety filters in dusty or fumy conditions are changed regularly
● reduce exposure to allergens such as pollen, dust or fur by not having pets, or 'trigger' plants in the garden
● use warm steam inhalations
● drink lots of fluid.

Tonsillitis and adenoidal conditions

Self help measures for these conditions include;
● bed rest
● plenty of fluids
● take analgesics such as paracetemol.

197

SUGGESTED FURTHER READING AND VIEWING

READING

BEES AND HONEY

'Bees - Lectures by Rudolf Steiner' translated from German by Thomas Braatz, ISBN 0-88010-457-0
Published by the Anthroposophic Press (1998)
3390 Route 9
Hudson, N.Y. 12534
USA

'Do you know about honeybees?' by Jennifer Buckle, ISBN 0-905652-30-4
Published by BBNO
Tapping Wall Farm
Burrowbridge
Somerset TA7 0RY

'Honey - Nature's secret weapon II (contained as section in book 'Vinegar - Nature's secret weapon') by Maxwell Stein, ISBN 0-9537074-7-4
Published by the Windsor Group (2002)
158 Moulsham Street
Chelmsford
Essex CM2 0LD

HAYFEVER

'Hayfever - How to cope with hayfever, asthma and related problems' by Dr. Jonathan Brostoff and Linda Gamlin, ISBN 0-7475-1699-5
Published by Bloomsbury Publishing Limited (1994)
2 Soho Square
London W1V 5DE

THE HISTORY OF MEDICINE

'The Greatest Benefit to Mankind' by Roy Porter, ISBN 0-00-637454-9
Published by Fontana Press an imprint of Harper Collins Publishers (1997)

'The History of Medicine' by Roberto Margotta, ISBN 0-7537-0541-9
Published by Chancellor Press (2001)

MÉNIÈRE'S DISEASE

'Vertigo and Dizziness' by Dr Lucy Yardley
Available from the website of the Ménière's Society: www.menieres.org.uk

MIGRAINE AND HEADACHE

'Coping Successfully with Migraine' by Sue Dyson
Published by Sheldon Press (fourth impression 1998) ISBN 0-85969-626-X
SPCK, Marylebone Road, London NW1 4DU

'The Migraine Handbook' by Jenny Lewis, ISBN 0-09-181666-1
C/o The Migraine Action Association
Unit 6, Oakley Hay Lodge Business Park
Great Folds Road,
Great Oakley, Northamptonshire NN18 9AS

'Migraine - understanding and coping with migraine' by Ann Rush
Published by Thorsons (1996), ISBN 0-7225-3265-2
C/o The Migraine Trust
55-56 Russell Square
London WC1B 4HP

'Hot Topics in Headache' Preface by Professor Peter J Goadsby
Available from the Migraine Trust
ISBN 0-9504-752-38

NATIVE NORTH AMERICANS
'Native North America - Belief and Ritual, Spirits of Earth and Sky' by Larry J.
Zimmerman, ISBN 1-903296-59-5
Published by Duncan Baird Publishers (DBP) 1996
6th Floor
Castle House
75 -76 Wells Street
London W1T 3QH

PRESSURE PROBLEMS
'Ears, Altitude and Airplane Travel'
American Academy of Otolaryngology brochure
Website: www.sinuscarecenter.com/bareraaoo.htlm

'A Survey of the Effects of Pressure on Ménière's Disease Symptoms'
by Dr Alec Salt (2000)
Website: Http://oto.wusl.edu/men/pressure/

SALT INTAKE
'Salt in Medical Practice'
Queensland Hypertension Association (Australia)
Email: armstrongr@gph.ramsayhealth.com.au

'Salt Matters: a consumer guide' by Trevor C Beard
Available from the Queensland Hypertension Association (Australia)
or from the Ménière's Society website www.menieres.org.uk

TINNITUS

'Tinnitus - Living with the ringing in your ears' by Richard Hallam
Published in the Thorsons Health Series, ISBN 0-7225-2940-6
3rd edition 1993
77 - 85 Fulham Palace Road
Hammersmith
London W6 8JB

'The Complete Guide to Tinnitus' by Maxwell Stein (2002)
Published by The Windsor Group Ltd, ISBN 1-903904-21-8
158 Moulsham Street
Chelmsford
Essex CM2 0LD

'Understanding Deafness and Tinnitus' by Professor Tony Wright
Published by Family Doctor Publications, ISBN 1-898205-98-1
Telephone 01202 668330 for mail order, Website: www.familydoctor.co.uk

'Understanding tinnitus - managing the noises in the ears or in your head' by Keith
Dunmore, Valerie Tait and Glynis Riddiford
Published for the RNID by Forest Books, ISBN 1-904296-02-5
Forest books Tel/ Text: 01594 833858, Email: forest@forestbooks.com
RNID shop: www.rnidshop.com

VIEWING

EAR CANDLING THERAPY

'A Guide to Ear Candling'
DVD format presented by Andrew Sceats
First in a series of complementary therapy videos
Purchase online from www.pressuredown.net
Accompanying music CD available.

EAR INFECTIONS AND GLUE EAR

'What You Really Need To Know about...Ear Infections and Glue Ear'
Video presented by Dr Robert Buckman and introduced by John Cleese
From a series 'Videos for Patients' available through The Production Tree
71 Masbro Road, London W14 0LS, United Kingdom
Telephone: 0207 610 5599   Fax: 0207 610 5333
Email: mail@productiontree.co.uk

MIGRAINE
'What You Really Need to Know about...Migraine'
Video presented by Dr Robert Buckman and introduced by John Cleese
From a series 'Videos for Patients' available through the Production Tree
Contact details shown above

EAR EXAMINATIONS
'Clinical Examination of the Ear (with ear pathologies)'
Video presented by Mr Edward Fisher
Available from the Institute of Laryngology & Otology
University College London
330/ 336 Gray's Inn Road
London WC1X 8EE
Telephone: 0207 915 1514 Fax: 0207 837 9279
Email: j.gibney@ucl.ac.uk

USEFUL ADDRESSES

ACOUSTIC NEUROMA
The British Neuroma Association
Oak House
Ransom Business Park
Southwell Road West
Mansfield
Nottinghamshire NG21 0HJ
United Kingdom
Telephone: 0800 652 3143
Website: www.ukan.co.uk Email: bana@ukan.freeserve.co.uk

CHINESE HERBAL MEDICINE
The Register of Chinese Herbal Medicine
Office 5, 1 Exeter Street
Norwich
Norfolk NR2 4QB
United Kingdom
Telephone: 01603 623994 Fax: 01603 667557
Website: www.rchm.co.uk Email: herbmed@rchm.co.uk
The RCHM was founded in 1987 and in a member of the European Herbal
Practitioners Association (EHPA)

COCHLEAR IMPLANTS
The National Cochlear Implant Users Association
PO Box 260
High Wycombe
Buckinghamshire HPII 1FA
United Kingdom
Website: www.nciua.demon.co.uk
Registered Charity No. 1073222

DEAF AND HARD OF HEARING PEOPLE
The Council for the Advancement of Communication with Deaf People
Durham University Science Park
Block 4, Stockton Road
Durham DH1 3UZ
United Kingdom
Telephone: 0191 383 1155, Text: 0191 383 7915, Fax: 0191 383 7914
Website: www.cacdp.org.uk, Email: durham@cacdp.org.uk
The CACDP is a registered UK charity (No. 1071662) whose main aim is to promote
communication between deaf, hard of hearing, deafblind and hearing people by
offering high quality nationally recognised assessments and accreditation in British
Sign Language (BSL) and other forms of communication used by deaf people.

Deafness Research UK
(formerly *Defeating Deafness (The Hearing Research Trust)*)
330/332 Gray's Inn Road
London WC1X 8EE
United Kingdom
Telephone: 0207 833 1733 Text: 0207 915 1412 Fax: 0207 278 0404
Website: www.deafnessresearch.org.uk Email: contact@deafnessresearch.org.uk

Deafness Research UK information service
Free phone: 0808 808 2222 Email: info@deafnessresearch.org.uk
Defeating Deafness is a research and education charity for hearing impaired people.
Registered Charity No. 326915

The National Deaf Children's Society (NDCS)
15 Dufferin Street
London EC1Y 8UR
United Kingdom
Telephone: 0207 490 8656 (voice/ fax), free phone helpline: 0808 800 8880 (v/ t)
Website: www.ndcs.org.uk Email: helpline@ndcs.org.uk
This Registered Charity (No.1016532), which was started in 1944, organises a wide
range of activities including parents' groups aimed at helping deaf children

The International Deaf Children's Society (IDCS)
15 Dufferin Street
London EC1Y 8UR
United Kingdom
Telephone: 0207 490 8656 Fax: 0207 251 5020
Website: www.idcs.info Email: idcs@idcs.info
The IDCS is the international arm of the NDCS (see above for details)

The Royal National Institute for Deaf and Hard of Hearing People (RNID)
19-23 Featherstone Street
London EC1Y 8SL
United Kingdom
Telephone: 0207 296 8000 Text: 0207 296 8001 Fax: 0207 296 8199
Website: www.rnid.org.uk Email: informationline@rnid.org.uk
RNID Helpline: PO Box 16464, London EC1Y 8TT
Telephone: 0870 60 50 123 Text: 0870 60 33 007
The RNID is a Registered Charity No. 207720

RNID Northern Ireland
Wilton House
5 College Square North
Belfast BT1 6AR
Northern Ireland
Telephone/ textphone: 02890 239619

RNID Scotland
Crown Gate Business Centre
Brook Street, Glasgow G40 3AP
Telephone: 0141 554 0053
Email: rnidscotland@rnid.org.uk

RNID Cymru (Wales)
Fourth Floor
16 Cathedral Road
Cardiff CF11 9LJ
Wales
Telephone: 029 2033 3034, Textphone: 029 2033 3036, Fax: 029 2033 3035
Email: rnidcymru@rnid.org.uk

GOLDENHAR SYNDROME
The Goldenhar Syndrome Family Support Group
Telephone: 0794 097 6327
Website: www.goldenhar.org.uk
The support group is a registered Charity No. 1099642 and has produced
'Parents Guide to Goldenhar Syndrome' (£4.00), 'Special Stories' (£6.00)

GOVERNMENT AGENCIES
The Health and Safety Executive
HSE Infoline
Caerphilly Business Park
Caerphilly
Wales CF83 3GG
Telephone: 08701 545500, Fax: 02920 859260, Minicom: 02920 808537
Website: www.hse.gov.uk   Email: hseinformationservices@natbrit.com
There are also information centres in London and Merseyside for personal callers.

LARYNGECTOMY
National Association of Laryngectomee Clubs
Lower Ground Floor
152 Buckingham Palace Road
Victoria
London SW1W 9TR
Telephone: 0207 730 8585 Fax: 0207 730 8585
website: www.nalc.ik.com

LIPREADING
The Association of Teachers of Lipreading to Adults
PO Box 506
Hanley
Stoke on Trent
Staffordshire ST2 9RE
United Kingdom
Email: atla@lipreading.org.uk

MÉNIÈRE'S DISEASE
Ménière's Society
The Rookery
Surrey Hills Business Park
Wotton, Surrey RH5 6QT
Telephone: 0845 120 2975 Minicom: 01306 876883 Fax: 01306 876057
Website: www.menieres.org.uk Email: info@menieres.org.uk

MIGRAINE
Migraine Action Association
Unit 6, Oakley Hay Lodge Business Park
Great Folds Road
Great Oakley
Northamptonshire NN18 9AS
United Kingdom
Telephone: 01536 461333 Fax: 01536 461444
Website: www.migraine.org.uk Email: info@migraine.org.uk
Registered Charity No. 207783

The Migraine Trust
55-56 Russell Square
London WC1B 4HP
United Kingdom
Telephone: 0207 436 1336 Fax: 0207 436 2880
Website: www.migrainetrust.org Email: info@migrainetrust.org
Registered Charity No. 1081300

SALT INTAKE
Salt Skip Programme
New South Wales Menieres Support Group (Australia)
www.hinet.net.au/~nswmsg/SaltSkip.htm

Queensland Hypertension Association (Australia)
PO Box 193 Holland Park
Queensland 4121
Australia
Telephone: (07) 3899 1659, Fax: (07) 3394 7815

SIGN LANGUAGE

Council for the Advancement of Communication with Deaf People (CACDP)
CACDP Head Office
Durham University Science Park
Block 4
Stockton Road
Durham DH1 3UZ
United Kingdom
Telephone: 0191 383 1155 (voice and text), Fax: 0191 383 7914
Website: www.cacdp.org.uk   Email: durham@cacdp.org.uk
The CACDP is the national examinations board for British Sign Language (BSL) examinations and give information about availability of BSL classes nationwide. BSL is the preferred language for over 70,000 deaf people; over 100,000 hearing people who have a proficiency in the language use it.

Visual Interpreting and Communication in Shropshire (VISS)
The Disability Resource Centre
Lancaster Road
Harlescott
Shrewsbury
Shropshire SY1 3NJ
United Kingdom
Telephone: 01743 440060, Minicom: 01743 440050, Fax: 01743 461349
Email: viss@shropshiredisability.org

SNORING AND SLEEP APNOEA

The British Snoring and Sleep Apnoea Association
Second Floor Suite
52 Albert Road North
Reigate
Surrey RH2 9EL.
Telephone: 0800 085 1097
Website: www.britishsnoring.co.uk
Email: admin@britishsnorting.co.uk

TINNITUS

British Tinnitus Association
Ground Floor, Unit 5
Acorn Business Park
Woodseats Close
Sheffield
South Yorkshire S8 0TB
United Kingdom
Telephone: 0800 018 0527; 0845 4500 321 (local rate); 0114 250 9933 (national rate). Fax: 0114 288 2279
Website: www.tinnitus.org.uk   Email: info@tinnitus.org.uk
The BTA is a Registered Charity No. 1011145

INDEX

squamous cell carcinoma 88
Tuning fork ear testing 70
Tyagi, B D 171
Tympanic (tympanum/ middle ear) cavity
45

Utricle 49,54

Vaccination 91,105
Valsalva's manoeuvre 84
Veins
    Carotid 41
    Jugular 41
Vertigo 78,110,191
    causes 78
    self help 93
    symptoms
    treatment
Vestibule 49
Vestibular system 53,131
Viruses 139
Vitamin B12 77,91
Vitamin C 142
Voice 35
    production 35
    transmission via facial skeleton 35

Warfarin 108
Waxsol 58
Western Herbalism 157
Willis, Thomas 125

X- rays 68,118,126,136